Healing
Immune Disorders

Healing Immune Disorders

Natural Defense Building Solutions

Allergy
Autoimmune Disease
Complementary Cancer Approaches
Chronic Fatigue
and More

Andrew Gaeddert

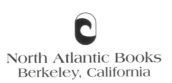

North Atlantic Books
Berkeley, California

Disclaimer

The following information is intended for general information purposes only. Individuals with a health problem should always see their health care provider before administering any suggestions made in this book. Any application of the material set forth in the following pages is at the reader's discretion and his or her sole responsibility.

Published by

North Atlantic Books
P.O. Box 12327
Berkeley, California 94712

Get Well Foundation
8001A Capwell Drive
Oakland, California 94621

Cover and book design by Catherine E. Campaigne
Distributed to the book trade by Publishers Group West
Printed in the United States of America

Healing Immune Disorders: Natural Defense Building Solutions is sponsored by the Society for the Study of Native Arts and Sciences, a nonprofit educational corporation whose goals are to develop an educational and crosscultural perspective linking various scientific, social, and artistic fields; to nurture a holistic view of arts, sciences, humanities, and healing; and to publish and distribute literature on the relationship of mind, body, and nature.

Healing Immune Disorders: Natural Defense Building Solutions is also sponsored by the Get Well Foundation, a nonprofit organization whose purpose is to educate the public and health care providers about natural therapies that are complements to Western medicine. Get Well Foundation operates a clinic, publishes books, and sponsors seminars.

Library of Congress Cataloging-in-Publication Data

Gaeddert, Andrew.
   Healing immune disorders : natural defense building solutions / by Andrew
Gaeddert.
      p. cm.
Summary: "Focuses on a natural approach to treating a variety of immune related
conditions through the use of Chinese and Western herbs and supplements, and
through changes in diet and lifestyle"—Provided by publisher.
Includes bibliographical references and index.
ISBN 1-55643-604-1 (pbk.)
   1. Immunologic diseases—Alternative treatment.   2. Herbs—Therapeutic
use.   3. Naturopathy. 4. Medicine, Chinese.   I. Title.
RC582.G34 2005
616.97'06—dc22

                                                            2005027131

*I would like to thank Carol Gaeddert
for her encouragement,
Misha Ruth Cohen, OMD, LAc for her inspiration,
and Laurie Dearborn for her editorial assistance.*

Table of Contents

List of Illustrations

Introduction

It can be challenging having an immune disorder, or having a loved one with an immune disorder. People are bombarded with chemicals and stress that our species has not adapted to, and it's wearing out our immune systems.

While many immune conditions aren't curable, they are treatable. People following the instructions in this book have been able to live a quality of life beyond what others thought was possible. In *Healing Immune Disorders,* we will focus on natural approaches. Improving immune function and treating autoimmune conditions involve: maximizing your digestive health, reducing stress, nourishing yourself with positive thoughts, and developing healthy habits.

There are several reasons to improve your immune system and put into action what is in this book: you will experience great energy levels and less fatigue, you will spend less time fighting infections, you will be able to recover faster if you do get sick, and finally you can help other people with immune and autoimmune conditions.

Herbs and lifestyle tips are presented to get you and your loved ones on the path to healing. Healing is more than getting rid of an illness. It is more than taking a promising herb or supplement or learning yoga. Healing is a discovery of the self. It is learning about what your body likes and what it does not like. Healing is exploring the best treatment plan, and how to combine the best of modern and natural medicine. It involves harnessing the healing force of nature, and learning how our immune health is influenced by our thoughts, our behaviors, and our environment.

If we think healthy thoughts, if we have supportive habits and relationships, if we contribute to others, we can make a healing journey no matter what the shape of our physical body. I use journey as a metaphor for healing because it is not always easy, and it is frequently not in a straight line; however, with focused intention you can get where you want to go. Therefore, it is essential when reading this book that you focus on "What do you want?" What are your goals, dreams, and desires independent of successfully treating your condition? If you were healthy what would you do?

Connie was sick and tried of being sick and tired. When I asked her what she wanted, Connie listed all the things she didn't want: *I'm tired of feeling run-down. I'm tired of being broke all the time. I don't want to be single all my life.* Therefore, her focus was all on being tired, broke, and single. What she wanted was improved energy reserves, a good income, and a good relationship. Once she could see clearly what she wanted, getting to the goal was much easier. Part of the work we did together was herbal and nutritional counseling; part of our work together was to help Connie move toward her dream of being a substance abuse counselor.

What are ten reasons you can think of to practice a healthier lifestyle? Did you know that some people can live happier and healthier lives after their diagnosis, than before they were diagnosed with a terminal illness? After he was diagnosed with Human Immunodeficiency Virus (HIV), Magic Johnson achieved a healthier lifestyle with more financial success than before his diagnosis. Superstar bicyclist Lance Armstrong went on to win the Tour de France seven times after he was given only a 10 percent chance of surviving his cancer diagnosis. In our clinic we have seen miracles from clients who are willing to participate fully in their health, and there is no reason why you can't live better than ever before.

In addition to lifestyle tips, we will discuss how to use herbs and supplements. Quality herbs are important because they promote vitality. Herbs can also be used to treat symptoms as well as drug side effects. Under the care of an experienced herbalist, it may be possible to treat the underlying imbalance that causes the symptoms you experience. The metaphor for biomedicine is "The disease was cured, but the patient died." The metaphor for natural medicine is "The soul was cured, and the patient thrived."

You will find herbal and nutritional supplements that can be self-administered and ones that require professional guidance. Whenever possible, we advise consulting an herbalist. When it comes to your own health, even the most highly trained practitioners seek the help of others. Why? It is very difficult to be objective about one's own health. A professional may be able to reach a different diagnosis than your medical doctor. They may have different explanations as to why you have symptoms and how you might heal.

For example, an herbalist trained in TCM (traditional Chinese medicine) might take into account your appearance. She might ask questions you have not thought of before like whether you prefer hot or cold, as well as questions about your perspiration, stools, and urination. You might be asked when your symptoms flare up. Typically your tongue and pulse are evaluated in different ways than in biomedicine.

3

In the best case, the herbalist may take into account your Western diagnosis, what she sees, and what she feels on your pulse in order to select the best herbs for your condition.

Herbal medicine has been with us for thousands of years. Today in the U.S. and elsewhere millions of people take herbs everyday. In the U.S., Europe, and Asia herbs are researched using modern techniques. As a rule herbs work more slowly and gently than drugs, and are better for maintaining the health of the immune system as they seldom have side effects. Western medical techniques such as drugs and surgery typically work best for the acute or crisis stage of immune disorders. In three clinical studies I have participated in, herbs were used along with Western drug protocols. In twenty years of practice, I can say the two systems are fully compatible.

In *Healing Immune Disorders* you'll find recommendations that will improve your quality of life no matter what your diagnosis. Whether you are someone with cancer or Acquired Immune Deficiency Syndrome (AIDS), or someone who gets too many colds or infections, following the exercises in the book and incorporating the best of conventional and complementary approaches will give you the potential to experience improved energy levels, more restful sleep, improved digestion, freedom from pain, and finally more inner peace.

How to use natural therapies: See a health professional who is trained in herbs and natural therapies whenever possible. Product quality can vary greatly. If you find a product that works for you keep using it. Generally products manufactured in the U.S. are made with more stringent quality controls than elsewhere. Failure to achieve results may indicate that you are not taking the correct remedy or the correct dosage. Make sure your goals are realistic. The goals of herbs and nutritional medicine are not to instantly cure illness. Herbs and other natural therapies work gradually to support the body's natural processes with fewer side effects than conventional drugs. You should allow at least a month of herbal therapy for every year you have had symptoms. Illnesses that are inherited (genetic) are usually more difficult to correct than illnesses that are acquired (that is, developed from bad diet or lifestyle choices). Don't put off medical appointments. Although there are many side effects from drugs and surgery, diagnostic tests may save your life. Natural approaches generally work best for chronic health problems whereas biomedical approaches may work better for acute health problems. If it sounds too good to be true—it probably is. Like biomedical approaches, instant results may also produce instant side effects or be overly expensive.

Chinese tradition view people with immune and autoimmune conditions according to their condition or temperature. Haven't you met people who run hot, or boil over at the slightest insult? Don't you know people who are always cold, when others are warm? Chinese medicine takes these constitutional factors into account before prescribing herbs or making dietary recommendations. Foods, as well as people, can be similarly classified. For example, chili peppers are warming and ice cream is cooling.

As an example of the principles of Chinese medicine, take the following two individuals; Megan is a thirty-two year old banker, diagnosed with Chronic Fatigue Syndrome (CFS), gets entirely different herbs than Williamina, forty-five, who has the same condition. Megan has what is considered a hot dry condition. She has afternoon fevers and fatigue, night sweats and exhaustion as she works too hard. Williamina has what is considered a cold type. She wakes up tired and gets increasingly exhausted as the day progresses. She often feels cold, she has loose stools, and swollen ankles.

I recommended that Megan take cooling herbs and special immune tonics. I suggested she drink peppermint tea as a beverage, as it has cooling properties. Williamina was counseled to take warming herbs and to eat and drink everything hot. I also recommend ginger tea, which has warming properties.

Below is a chart for you to access your basic constitution; dietary and lifestyle suggestions included.

Hot and Dry Conditions	Dampness	Cold
◆ Sensations of heat	◆ Swelling or edema	◆ Sensations of coldness
◆ Symptoms worse with hot weather	◆ Mucus	◆ Condition worsens in winter
◆ Bright red papules or macules	◆ Food allergies	◆ Excessive urination
◆ Smoking	◆ Symptoms worse in moldy damp environments	◆ Dry skin (blood deficiency)
◆ Easily angered	◆ Intestinal gas, bloating, indigestion	◆ Itching worse in cold
◆ Constipation (can also be due to cold)	◆ Pulse, sluggish	◆ History of anemia
◆ Easily upset	◆ Sadness or depression (feeling weighted down)	◆ Chronic loose stools
◆ Prone to afternoon slump	◆ Worry	◆ Tongue, pale
◆ Dark urine	◆ Dull sensations	◆ Pulse, slow and sinking
◆ Loud and dominating	◆ Food intolerance	
◆ Yellow phlegm	◆ Hay fever	
◆ Fast pulse rate	◆ Tongue, pale with thick coating	
◆ Early and heavy menstruation, bright red blood	◆ Pulse, slippery quality	
◆ Burning and dryness of the skin		
◆ Thirst		
◆ Tongue, red and dry		
◆ Pulse, rapid and may be floating		

Note to Practitioners

Healing Immune Disorders is designed for both practitioners and laypeople. It encourages laypeople to see a trained herbalist whenever possible as self-treatment can be difficult, especially for chronic and terminal diseases. One of my concerns treating people twenty years ago, was whether use of immune tonic herbs could worsen an autoimmune condition. In almost every case, we have seen appropriately recommended herbs benefit people with immune and autoimmune conditions. Of course, in every case it is essential to assess the strength of the pathogen, in connection with the strength of the individual's constitution. Although this book uses mostly Western terminology, I believe that the best way to evaluate an individual's constitution is by keeping in mind the pulse, the tongue, and the eight principles of diagnosis along with the twenty questions used in TCM (traditional Chinese medicine). For more information on diagnosis please see my book *Chinese Herbs in the Western Clinic*. For more information about the individual herbs contained in the formulas please see *Chinese Herbal Medicine: Materia Medica* by Dan Bensky, Steven Clavey, and Erich Stöger, with Andrew Gamble.

How to Use Natural Therapies

1. See a health professional who is trained in herbs and natural therapies whenever possible.
2. Product quality can vary greatly. If you find a product that works for you keep using it. Generally products manufactured in the U.S. are made with more stringent quality controls than elsewhere.
3. Failure to achieve results may indicate that you are not taking the correct remedy or the correct dosage.
4. Make sure your goals are realistic. The goals of herbs and nutritional medicine are not to instantly cure illness. Herbs and other natural therapies work gradually to support the body's natural processes with fewer side effects than conventional drugs. You should allow at least a month of herbal therapy for every year you have had symptoms.
5. Illnesses that are inherited (genetic) are usually more difficult to correct than illnesses that are acquired (that is, developed from bad diet or lifestyle choices).
6. Don't put off medical appointments. Although there are many side effects from drugs and surgery, diagnostic tests may save your life. Natural approaches generally work best for chronic health problems whereas biomedical approaches may work better for acute health problems.
7. If it sounds too good to be true—it probably is. Like biomedical approaches, instant results may also produce instant side effects or be overly expensive.

Chapter One

Tips for a Healthy Immune System

Learn About Your Immune System

Your immune system's main job is to protect you from infection and cancer. Our bodies have an innate, nonspecific immune response that acts on any outside invaders, and a learned immune response through which our immune system learns to act more quickly and powerfully when it sees a specific antigen a second time. This learned immunity explains why vaccines work, and why people don't get chickenpox or measles twice.

There are two basic types of immune problems. A deficient immune system leaves the body open to attack from the outside, while in autoimmune disease, the immune system mistakenly attacks the body itself. If your immune system is weak, you may be plagued by frequent, lingering colds and other infections. Cancer develops partially because the immune system fails to recognize cancer cells as a threat, and thus fails to activate an immune response. In autoimmune conditions, the body mistakes its own tissues for invaders, and attacks itself. In the case of allergies, the immune system overreacts to an allergen that doesn't actually present an immediate danger to the body.

Immune Deficiency

When the immune system malfunctions, the body is vulnerable to the countless microbes surrounding us and living inside us. AIDS, in which the human immunodeficiency virus (HIV) kills the T cells that make the immune response happen, has made us all aware of the importance of a healthy immune system. Hodgkin's disease, cancer of the lymph nodes, can suppress lymph node cells. Chemotherapy drugs used to treat cancer also suppress the immune system. Our lifestyle choices can suppress our immune systems; choices like drinking a lot of alcohol, eating junk food, exercising excessively, and smoking. Stress, whether emotional or physical, suppresses the immune system in a number of ways. Macrophages, for example, become sluggish when you're depressed. Stress releases cortisol and epinephrine, which then suppress T cells. Stress makes everything worse—for example, a number of classic studies show that students cramming for exams are more likely to come down with a cold. Allergies, infections, surgery, radiation, and drugs also suppress the immune system. Herbs, good sleep, a healthy diet, a positive attitude, friends and family, community ties, moderate exercise, recreation, and music can boost the immune system.

Autoimmune Disease

The major histocompatibility complex (MHC) is a group of protein molecules found on the surface of all our cells that identify our tissues as our own, and not some foreign invader. The immune system normally knows what to attack and what to leave alone. It spares, for example, the beneficial bacteria that help digestion. It usually knows not to attack the food you eat, or a developing fetus. In autoimmune diseases, the immune system can't differentiate between the self and the nonself, and mistakenly attacks the cells, tissues, and organs of the body as if they were dangerous invaders.

Different autoimmune diseases affect different parts of the body. For example, Crohn's disease and ulcerative colitis attack the gastrointestinal system, psoriasis affects the skin, and Hashimoto's thyroiditis attacks the thyroid. Autoimmune diseases often attack multiple systems in the body, so symptoms can be confusing and diagnosis difficult. Because there's no medical specialty in autoimmune disease, people with autoimmune disorders end up seeing a long list of specialists: a dermatologist for skin symptoms, a rheumatologist for joint pain, an endocrinologist for hormonal issues. Autoimmune disease, in general, often runs in families, though usually not the same autoimmune disease.

Women are hit harder by autoimmune disorders than men. Of the estimated fifty million people in the U.S. affected by the eighty-plus chronic, disabling conditions recognized as autoimmune in nature, 75–90 percent are women. It hasn't been proven exactly how, but hormones, particularly estrogens and androgens, are thought to be responsible for this gender difference. Autoimmune disease symptoms in women often get better or worse with changes in hormone levels—for example, during pregnancy or after menopause. Because women are designed to carry a baby for nine months, the female immune system is more complex and sensitive than the male immune system, which only has to deal with fighting off outside pathogens. Women with autoimmune disorders tend to have high estrogen levels, and tend to improve when their estrogen levels drop at menopause. In men, on the other hand, autoimmune problems increase as they age, when androgen levels decrease and estrogen levels relatively increase.

Female/Male Ratios in Autoimmune Disease[1]

Hashimoto's disease/hypothyroiditis	50:1
Systemic lupus erythematosus	9:1
Sjögren's syndrome	9:1
Antiphospholipid syndrome	9:1
Primary biliary cirrhosis	9:1
Mixed connective tissue disease	8:1
Chronic active hepatitis	8:1
Graves' disease/hyperthyroiditis	7:1
Rheumatoid arthritis	4:1
Scleroderma	3:1
Myasthenia gravis	2:1
Multiple sclerosis	2:1
Chronic idiopathic thrombocytopenic purpurea	2:1

Inflammatory Response

Inflammation is a healing response triggered by any injury to body tissues, whether due to a physical trauma or to an infection.

Following the injury, immune cells make chemicals that promote dilation of capillaries, the smallest blood vessels. With more blood flowing to the area, it gets red and hot. These chemicals also make the capillaries more permeable, allowing antibodies and clotting proteins to seep from the capillaries into surrounding tissue, causing swelling, called edema, which presses on nerves, causing pain. This swelling, though it hurts, actually promotes the healing process by bringing helpful immune cells to the site. Fever happens when an infection is more widespread, and like inflammation, also speeds up healing processes. Inflammation is at work in many autoimmune illnesses, but instead of helping the body to heal, it is out of control, continually attacking the body and causing pain and disease.

Immunity in TCM

In Chinese, immunity translates as mian yi. Mian means "protect" and yi means "epidemic diseases." The term mian yi first appeared in Chinese medical literature in the 18th century, but the concept goes back at least two thousand years, when the *Yellow Emperor's Classic of Medicine,*[2] an early medical text, stated, "If the body is full of vital energy (Qi), it will not be invaded by pathogens."

Immunization is thought to go back more than a thousand years in Chinese medicine, as documented in *A Handbook for Prescriptions for Emergencies,* or *Zhou Hou Bei Ji Fang,* which recommended preventing rabies by applying powder from an infected dog to the bite. The Chinese also used inoculations to prevent smallpox in the 16th century. And according to a 17th century Chinese text called *Readings for Medical Professionals,* or *Yi Zong Bi Du,* tumors are caused by weak vital energy, or Qi, just as cancer is today considered to arise from suppressed immune function.

In Chinese medicine terms, immunity and health depend on both inherited, constitutional Qi, also called original Qi, and acquired Qi. While some people are blessed with hardy genes, or plentiful original Qi, acquired Qi is even more important to your immune health, and fortunately is easily enhanced by eating well, getting restful sleep, minimizing stress, and engaging in fun, healthy activities such as physical exercise.

The spleen and kidney are the two organ systems most associated with original Qi and thus with the immune system. Studies have shown that patients with spleen deficiency, in Chinese medicine terms, also have low T-lymphocyte counts and lower levels of the immunoglobulins IgA and IgG. Chinese herbal treatments can return these lab values to normal. Patients diagnosed as kidney deficient by a Chinese medicine practitioner show more profound reductions in IgA and IgG, and may also have IgE reactions that trigger inflammation. Treatment with kidney tonic herbs tends to reduce IgE levels and increase T-helper cells.[3]

In Chinese medicine terms, a weak immune system is also seen as a deficiency of defensive Qi, or wei qi. Wei qi is the Qi that circulates at the very surface of the skin, where it warms the skin and muscles and protects against exterior pathogenic factors. The lung system is responsible for dispersing the wei qi throughout the body, so if the lung qi is deficient, the wei qi won't be dispersed adequately, leaving us open to colds and infections. The Qi that protects the body from invasion by exterior pathogenic factors is also called zheng qi, which translates as upright qi or righteous qi. These terms are usually used in reference to a pathogen, indicating the degree of resistance to disease.

The Invaders

An antigen is any substance that triggers an immune response. We live in a world teeming with bacteria, viruses, fungi, and parasites, which can cause us much grief if our immune system is weak and can't fight them off. The immune system's job is to protect the body from foreign invaders, or external evils as we say in Chinese medicine. When the immune system recognizes bacteria, viruses, parasites, cancer cells, or transplanted tissues and organs as outsiders, it triggers the immune response. If the immune system is weak and unable to muster the necessary resources, we get an infection, or a cold, or a more serious illness.

Bacteria are single-celled organisms, some of which can cause disease either by directly killing cells or with their toxic waste products. Common bacteria that cause illness include staphylococci, streptococci, chlamydia, gonococci, and rickettsia. Most bacteria, however, are not harmful. The good ones are called probiotics. Acidophilus, is an example, which lives in the intestine, where it helps with digestion and controls overgrowth of harmful bacteria.

Viruses are parasitic—they need to get into your body's cells to live and reproduce. To reproduce, they must take over a cell and use its DNA. The common cold, influenza, polio, and AIDS are all caused by a virus.

Fungi are single-celled organisms—including molds, yeasts, and mushrooms—that look and act a lot like plants. There are thousands of kinds of fungus, about one hundred of which may cause disease, including athlete's foot and ringworm. Candida is a common fungus that causes thrush and vaginal yeast infections.

Parasites are single-celled organisms that get into the body and live there. Malaria and giardia are two well-known diseases caused by protozoan parasites. The larger parasitic worms, also called helminths, enter the body and live off nutrients found in the intestines, lungs, liver, skin, and brain. The most common parasitic worms include tapeworms, roundworms, and hookworms.

The Immune Players

Mucous membranes are on the front line when it comes to fighting off infectious invaders. For example, the hairs in your nose and the tiny hair-like cilia in your respiratory tract, both act to filter out invaders. Mucous membrane secretions like tears, saliva, skin oils, and stomach acid all contain bacteria-killing substances.

Lymph is a milky fluid made of immune white blood cells and fat. Lymph circulates throughout the body in lymphatic vessels, to lymph nodes found under the arms, behind the ears, and in the groin, where antigens and cellular debris are eaten up by special cells called macrophages before the lymph is returned to the blood.

Bone marrow produces the stem cells that make red blood cells and most immune cells.

The thymus is a butterfly-shaped gland lying below the thyroid and above the heart. The thymus is a major gland of the immune system, and people with impaired immune function usually have impaired thymus function. The thymus makes T cells, which are responsible for cell-mediated immunity. Cell-mediated immunity includes immune functions that don't involve antibodies, and is important in resistance to bacteria, yeast, fungi, parasites, and viruses, as well as in protecting against cancer and autoimmune disorders. The thymus also releases hormones that regulate immune functions, including thymosin, thymopoietin, and serum thymic factor. Thymic hormone levels are often low in people who are prone to infection, in cancer and AIDS patients, and in the elderly.

The spleen, located in the upper left abdomen behind the stomach, is the largest lymph system organ. The spleen makes lymphocytes and cleans the blood, removing toxins and harmful microbes from the blood. It also makes immune-enhancing proteins such as tuftsin and splenopentin.

White Blood Cells

The many different types of white blood cells (WBCs) are key players in the immune system. The phagocytes (phago means "eat") are the first immune cells to greet pathogens that get past the mucosa or under your skin. Phagocytes eat harmful cells by surrounding them like an amoeba engulfs its food, and then releasing various chemicals to kill the cells. Macrophages, a type of phagocyte whose name means literally "big eaters," are the largest of the phagocytes. They not only eat pathogens but also send information about the harmful cells to other immune cells. Neutrophils, the most numerous of the phagocytes, destroy bacteria, tumor cells, and dead cells and are particularly important in preventing bacterial infection. Eosinophils and basophils secrete histamine and other substances that destroy antigens but also cause allergic reactions.

Lymphocytes are a type of WBC found in the lymph nodes, tonsils, bone, marrow, spleen, liver, lungs, and intestines, and are always ready to launch an immune response. There are three types of lymphocytes: B cells, named for their origin in bone marrow; T cells (also known as CD cells), named for their origin in the thymus gland; and natural killer cells.

T cells coordinate the immune response by interacting with the major histocompatibility complex to identify antigens. The three types of T cells have distinct functions. Killer T cells destroy cancer, viruses, and foreign tissue; helper T cells stimulate B cells to make antibodies; and suppressor T cells tell the B cells to stop making antibodies. HIV, for example, cripples the immune system by attacking helper T cells, which is why HIV-positive patients' T cell counts are closely monitored.

When they get signals from cytokines sent by T cells, B cells make antibodies, also called immunoglobulins, and attach them to invading antigens. The antibodies, in turn, alert other immune cells that the antigens are dangerous and need to be destroyed, and also help the body remember this invader for future reference.

Natural killer (NK) cells police the body, and are unique in that they can kill cancer and virus cells before the immune system responds to the invaders. They're called "natural" killers because they can kill any pathogenic cell, not just those that have already been "tagged" by the B cells. NK cells also produce interferon, which prevents viruses from reproducing. NK cells are particularly active in controlling cancer—people with high NK activity levels are less vulnerable to cancer and other illnesses, while those with low NK activity are more likely to get cancer, particularly metastatic cancer.

NK cells also produce cytokines, which are the messengers of the immune system. There are many types of cytokines, but among the most familiar are interferons, which prompt cells to make virus-killing enzymes; interleukins, which activate immune cells; growth factors, which help to heal injured tissues; and tumor necrosis factor, which kills cancer cells and shrinks tumors by cutting off their blood supply. Interferons are so named because they stimulate a chemical that interferes with virus reproduction. Interferons are special because they're not specific, but protect against a variety of viruses. They activate macrophages and NK cells, both of which act against cancer cells. Interferon is currently used as a treatment for genital warts, hepatitis C, and Kaposi's sarcoma. Substances that block tumor necrosis factor are being used to treat conditions including Crohn's disease and rheumatoid arthritis.

Complement proteins complement, or enhance, the immune response and also kill bacteria. Complement proteins are a group of twenty plasma proteins—including C1 through C9 and factors B, D, and P—that circulate inactive in the blood until activated by the immune response, or by interactions between factors B, D, and P with polysaccharide molecules on the surface of certain microorganisms. Complement proteins also stimulate mast cells and basophils to release histamine, which in turn attracts neutrophils and other immune cells to the area.

Immunoglobulins

Immunoglobulins, also called antibodies, are proteins made by B cells and plasma cells in response to an antigen. They protect the body by binding to antigens, and flagging them for destruction by other immune cells. Viral infections, radiation, and toxins can all cause an acquired immune deficiency, which is commonly treated with injections of gamma globulin, the part of the blood that contains immunoglobulins. There are five major types of immunoglobulin with different roles and locations in the body.

- **IgA** is found in the body's secretions, such as saliva, tears, and mucus. It's on the front line protecting the body's mucous membranes, including the walls of the gastrointestinal tract.
- **IgM** is the first antibody to respond to a new infection.
- **IgG** is the most common immunoglobulin, found throughout the body. IgG is activated later in the immune response, so its presence indicates a more established infection.
- **IgE** is the antibody at work in allergic reactions. It causes mast cells and basophils to release histamines, which fight

large invaders like parasites. When it responds inappropriately to harmless allergens, you get allergy symptoms.
- **IgD** is found on the outside of B cells, and it identifies foreign antigens.

Decide to Heal

For some of us, getting healthy is a scary proposition. Change means uncertainty, and uncertainty is uncomfortable. Before embarking on a new healing regime, I suggest seriously considering whether you are really ready to heal, and ready to make the changes necessary to do so. If you are willing to do whatever it takes, your potential is limitless.

Healing often takes time and is not always easy. Healing may require taking medications or herbs regularly, following through on lifestyle and dietary advice, and charting your progress mentally or by keeping a journal. Whatever the therapy, follow-through is extremely important. If you don't like your practitioner, or trust that they are looking out for your best interests, it's fine to see someone else. But it is essential that you follow your health professional's advice. Before trying a new approach, ask yourself, "Did I follow my last doctor's advice fully?" If you find yourself starting a lot of programs and not seeing sufficient benefit, you might ask yourself, "Am I ready to heal?" Although you might assume that anybody going to a health professional wants to see improvement, not everyone is ready or willing to do what it takes to see that improvement.

Our client Jeffery had been diagnosed with chronic fatigue syndrome and fibromyalgia. He had little energy during the day, slept poorly at night, and had pain all over his body. Jeffery went to several medical specialists, as well as several complementary providers. He tried acupuncture off and on, went to a chiropractor a few times, and was experimenting with a new kind of injection with a holistic doctor, but he found it all too expensive. When Jeffery came to our clinic, we told him that the herbs and supplements we recommended would most likely help many of his symptoms, but he would have to come to our clinic every week or every two weeks so we could monitor him. Part of the reason we do this is to avoid herb-drug interactions, and partly it's so we can evaluate the response to the herbs and supplements to see if adjustments are necessary.

Although Jeffery was supposed to come in every week or every two weeks, he ended up coming in every three weeks or every month. While he had seen some progress with our recommendations, he questioned the formulas we recommended compared with those dispensed by his chiropractor. Although we specialize in knowing which herbs and supplements would help him the most, he preferred to shop for the cheapest sources. While we pointed out that for the program we planned for him to work, he would have to be more faithful, he always had excuses, and after three months, we did not see Jeffery again.

Paul, on the other hand, an HIV patient with many of the same symptoms as Jeffery, took the opposite approach with excellent results. He came in for his regular appointments, he followed through on our program, frequently asking if there was anything he could do to gain additional progress, and he improved dramatically.

Illness can become a habit. The longer we are sick, the more ingrained the habit. Healthy people have habits that keep them healthy. They get up, eat, go to work, and have healthy habits that help relieve stress. Many of my clients, however, have habits that don't work for them. The first thing they do every morning when they wake up is to scan their body for what hurts. After they have done an inventory of all their aches and pains, they stew on it for a couple of hours. Throughout the day, they update their catalog of what isn't fair, what hurts. They are in the habit of thinking things like, "It's never going to get better." "Nothing works." "If only the pain would go away." Much of their day is spent in this habit of avoidance. If you asked these people what's good about being sick, they'd tell you there's nothing good about being sick.

Sue was a fifty-year-old woman who had been dealing with the symptoms of chronic fatigue syndrome for about ten years. She woke up tired after twelve hours in bed, and if she didn't get her midday nap, she couldn't function at all. Despite her fatigue, Sue had a lot to be thankful for. She was attractive, she had many interests, and three boys—two in college, and one in high school—all doing well. She had been married to her high school sweetheart for thirty years, and her husband, who drove her to her appointment in our clinic, seemed like a very lovable person. At our appointment, we recommended that she take an herbal decoction, as well as an herbal formula in tablet form. While in the office, she said she was willing to "do whatever it takes." Because she had to come a great distance to see me, I suggested she come every two weeks, although ideally I like to see a person the first week after beginning to take herbs. I pointed out that it would be necessary to come every two weeks if she really wanted to get better. She agreed.

Three days after her appointment, she left two messages on my answering machine. One message said that she needed to reschedule her appointment; she couldn't come back in two weeks; her other message was that she noticed that whenever she *didn't* take the tea, she felt tired. This raised two questions in my mind. Why was she—after only three days—rescheduling her appointment? And why was she not taking the tea as directed?

When I look at clients like Sue, I see someone whose illness provides her with certain advantages. Because she's sick, she doesn't have to work. Because she is easily confused, her husband or son chauffeured her around. Because she had an accident in the supermarket three years ago, her husband does most of the family shopping. My intention is not to pick on Sue here, but to make the point that in order to feel healthier, you need to act healthier.

Focus on the Positive

In the Navajo tradition children are taught that every morning when the sun comes up, it's a new sun. Resenting and complaining and worrying are a refusal to see how wonderful and precious life is. We can get so caught up in our own personal pain or worries that we don't notice that the wind has come up or that somebody has put flowers on the dining room table. Resentment, bitterness, and holding a grudge prevent us from seeing and hearing and tasting and delighting.

To heal your immune system, look toward a future in which you are healthy. As motivational speaker Anthony Robbins says, "Your past does not equal your future." The more positive you feel about your future, the less worry and discontent you will experience, and the healthier your immune system will be. The great American writer Ralph Waldo Emerson said, "A man is what he thinks about all day long." It's important to anticipate a future that is productive for yourself and for others. All too often, those of us with a chronic disease focus too much on the next hospital visit, or a feeling that we are being picked on.

Those who overcome chronic disease refuse to be victims. When asked about his colon cancer, Ronald Reagan replied, "I didn't have cancer, I had something inside me that had cancer inside it, and it was removed." Turn away from your fears and move toward your desires. Many of us fear never-ending pain, hospitalization, even death, while we desire health and a more productive life for ourselves and our families. See yourself in your mind's eye as being well, doing healthy things for yourself and others, and above all, constantly remind yourself of what is working well in your life. Many of the physically handicapped people I have worked with are remarkably optimistic. Be thankful for the ability to see, hear, think, taste, dream, and have a spouse, friends, and family. We often forget to appreciate the small but precious things.

> If you have a health challenge, decide how you want to feel. Then, figure out what stops you from feeling the way you want to feel. Decide what you are willing to do differently. What alternatives do you have? What would feeling differently do for you? Then, identify your first step toward feeling the way you want to feel.

Suffering is holding onto the negative aspects of our situation. Even a small problem can become insurmountable if we constantly think about how unfair it is or how much we are in pain. Positive thoughts and actions can help you separate the pain from the suffering. Try to think of thoughts as if you were a fish watching hooks dangling from the surface. Some of the hooks are temptations to dwell in the darkness of our moods, our despair, while others are invitations to think positively. You can choose your thoughts. You can watch your thoughts bobbing about without getting hooked by them. When you learn to not see your problems through a negative filter, you can be more positive about everything. Occupy your mind and body by exercising, reading, drawing, playing music, or gardening to keep your mind at bay.

It's easy to feel a lack of confidence, because many of us were raised without much adult support. When children are neglected, they suffer from a lack of encouragement. Children growing up in a single- or two-parent household may not get enough encouragement. Mom or dad may mean well, but they buy into the old saying

"Spare the rod and spoil the child." Others may feel that encouragement and praise might spoil the child. Some parents are excessively demanding. When Mike was growing up, his parents insisted he get straight As, and he was actually punished if he got a B.

A powerful remedy to low confidence is to realize that, given who you are, how you were raised, you did the best you could with the situation you had. Rather than work or wait for a future situation where you can feel happy, what can you feel good about right now? For a former prisoner, it may be being out of prison, or even being able to see natural light. How have you imprisoned yourself with negative chatter, a bleak worldview? How do you think your immune system responds? The immune system reflects our own inner states. Studies show that people who are optimistic and learn how to respond appropriately to stress are much less likely to become ill, and they heal more quickly if they do become sick.

The best metaphor for healing is that of a journey. Like a long trip, not all moments are pleasant, but looking back, it was worth the effort. Part of the healing journey involves having days when you don't feel 100 percent, and days when you feel like you're not making any progress at all. When you have these feelings, the first thing to do is relax and breathe. When you're feeling calmer, look at all the changes you've made since embarking on your healing journey. It's important that you get good at encouraging yourself. Find phrases that are particularly meaningful or helpful to you, such as "Good job, way to go."

Tips and Affirming Changes

Ask yourself:

- What am I happy about in my life now?
- Who do I love?
- Who loves me?
- What am I grateful about?

Find the Good in Your Illness

Optimism and hope speed recovery from illness. The more you can relax and find appreciation, the better your body will be able to heal itself. Any illness gives us a chance to slow down and appreciate life. There can be moments of meaning and pleasure, even in the midst of our suffering. What can you feel good about? Can you read a good book, pray, or meditate? Could you call or write someone that you haven't made the time to connect with in awhile? What about listening to the sounds outside your window? Can you watch how the light makes patterns on the ground? Could you spend time looking at a candle, picture, or flower?

When Cindy was hospitalized for a life-threatening infection, she was grateful that she had friends and family to call and visit her in the hospital. For the first time in months, she had the opportunity to read the newspaper and watch comedies she would never watch if she wasn't sick.

"I looked at being HIV-positive as an opportunity to change my whole life," said Ron, "and it has been exactly that. I am much healthier now than before I was diagnosed." When Ron was diagnosed with HIV, he did everything he could to improve his health. He dumped his friends who spent all their time drinking and partying, and he joined a gym where he made new friends who had healthy habits. As a medical school dropout, he believed in alternative medicine, and when one of his new friends suggested he see a local acupuncturist, he was open to trying it. The acupuncturist recommended an herbal formula, which seemed to give him more energy. He was heartened that the acupuncturist didn't tell him to stop all his medications, but selected a program of acupuncture and herbs to support his body, and suggested he enroll in a tai chi class, where he met even more new positive friends.

Many of us overlook the positive things in our life, but emphasize the negative. When first diagnosed with Multiple Sclerosis (MS), Daisy developed all the classic signs and symptoms. She was extremely depressed, and found it difficult to get out of bed. She kept remembering her grandmother, who also had MS. As a young girl, Daisy was responsible for cleaning up the mess when her grandmother wet the bed. Daisy kept remembering the lingering smell of unwashed urine on her grandmother's sheets and legs. She remembered her grandmother hobbling around the house, and the frequent falls.

One day, Daisy's minister came to visit her at home. The minister told her that many of the members of her church really missed her, and wouldn't it be wonderful if she could make it to church the next week. Although she didn't feel like it, she allowed her husband to get out the wheelchair and take her to church.

The sun was bright, a friend from church gave her flowers, and there was much joy and warmth. Another friend from church had great results at our clinic, and suggested that Daisy see us. Daisy came in shortly after her visit to church. I told her about a friend's wife, who had done well with her disease because soon after the MS diagnosis, she decided to help others rather than wallow in her condition. I advised Daisy to make images in her mind of some of her favorite times in life, and pleasant smells of her favorite flowers. And to use those images played on a big movie screen, to replace the unpleasant memories of her grandmother's illness, and the unpleasant smells, which she could shrink into a little black-and-white TV. We also suggested herbs and acupuncture, and a special yoga class for the disabled. On following visits, I suggested she stretch her mind to include seeing movie screen images of herself getting out of her wheelchair. Within three months, Daisy was out of the wheelchair. She felt much better, taking the herbs, going to acupuncture, and the special yoga class. She was also going to church again, every Sunday, and even helping to teach some of the kids in Sunday school.

Treat Yourself as a Friend

In order to mobilize your physical strength, it's important that your psychology is working with you and your immune system, rather than against you. People with autoimmune diseases are often self-critical. People who heal, on the other hand, believe in themselves more than they believe in the odds, or doctors, or science. People who heal realize that statistics have to do with averages, and that they are anything but average.

The Bible says to "love thy neighbor as thyself." In other words, not only is it important to love our neighbor, but it's also important to love ourselves. Unfortunately, self-love is generally associated with solipsism, conceit, and egotism, and is far from what most people actually feel about themselves.

How could you treat yourself more as a friend? What nice thing could you do for yourself? Could you buy yourself a treat? Give yourself a hug? Believe in yourself? Take a lemon balm tea bath?

Think about appreciating yourself. What do you like about yourself? What have you done for yourself and others lately? If nothing comes to mind, ask yourself what you could do for yourself or others. What about giving someone a compliment? While you're at it, what about giving yourself a compliment? Are you a hard worker? You could commend a friend for being a hard worker; what about commending yourself? Do you know how to have a good time? Being able to enjoy yourself and have fun is a valuable life skill—we weren't put on the planet to suffer.

Think about the things you've complimented others about.

Their appearance? What about your favorite article of clothing? Can you compliment yourself about the way you feel in that clothing? Did you leave a waitress a big tip? You should be commended.

How does your favorite person view you? Take a moment to see yourself through your favorite person's eyes. What do they see in you? Did you have a favorite relative when you were growing up, someone who was always supportive? What did they see in you? What do they see in you now? If they are no longer alive, what do you imagine they see in you? How can you begin to take an interest in yourself?

Self-appreciation is not about trying to get rid of all our bad qualities, or about ignoring them, but about noticing the good and the bad, and knowing you probably did a pretty good job all along, being raised the way you were, coming from the environment you did, and having the experiences you had. It is not at all about being selfish—in fact, it's just the opposite, because by learning to appreciate ourselves, we can better appreciate other people. Can you watch yourself criticize, get upset with, and be angry with yourself, but can you make friends with yourself knowing that you are not, nor will you ever be, perfect?

It's important to recognize your positive qualities, and to appreciate any small steps you make on your healing journey. Concentrating on appreciating is a way to tune out life's unpleasant distractions and annoyances. For example, if someone cuts you off on the freeway on the way to work, it's easy to get upset, but if you're busy appreciating the beautiful day, you're less likely to let it get you all worked up. Isn't it wonderful to drive to work, instead of having to walk in the rain? Isn't it wonderful to have a job to go to? When asked what was good about chronic pain, a Tibetan monk responded that it is such a wonderful thing to have a human body—and to be able to feel at all!

Traits of People Who Overcome Serious Medical Conditions

- They consider themselves fortunate, and are incredibly grateful for every day they are alive.
- They don't sweat the small stuff.
- They have a sense of purpose, a broader vision that prevents them from getting derailed by temporary setbacks.
- They believe in a higher power.
- They are fighters, and will do whatever it takes.
- They are not in denial. People who heal accept their condition, and then come up with a plan of attack for addressing it directly.
- They participate in their own recovery. They're proactive in their relationships with health professionals and persistent in trying alternative treatments. They know which symptoms to ignore and when to see a professional, when to get a second opinion, and when to seek alternative medicine.
- They don't accept "sentences." When she was told, "You have six months to live," Gloria told her doctor, "F*#$ you!"
- They focus on positive goals, and avoid dwelling on hardships.
- They are dedicated to regaining full strength.
- They take one step at a time, concentrating on a single task in the present moment, and celebrate milestones along the way.
- They don't compare themselves to others, but focus on their own progress, and celebrate how far they've come since last week, last month, and last year.

Get Rid of the ANTs

Most of us are constantly barraged by negative thoughts, worries, and emotions, chattering endlessly at us. For example, we may be bombarded with, *"Will I always be sick and tired? I used to have more energy. How will I ever make it to my son's wedding? . . . I wonder if they will even miss me when I'm dead. . . . What if I try alternative treatments and they don't work? . . ."*

By making an effort to reduce the negative chatter, we can help ourselves to heal. For example, positive chatter might sound something like: *"I'm glad I have a wife and three kids. . . . Maybe the herbs and supplements are working. . . . I wonder if I should go see the acupuncturist for pain control. . . . It sure helped my friend Hank."*

It's important to fill one's conscious and subconscious mind with positive self-talk. One of my clients, Carl, told me, "I always worry. My life should be perfect. I just got married, my career is going well, I don't even work very hard, but I'm constantly worrying!" My advice was to get the ANTs out of his head. ANTs stands for Automatic Negative Thoughts. Your head is filled with old "tapes" inserted by people in your past, such as your parents or other authority figures. I recommended that he start listening to progressive relaxation and self-hypnosis tapes. When he needed to refocus on the positive, I suggested he try asking himself: *What am I happy about in my life now? Who do I love? Who loves me? What am I grateful about?*

A technique I use every night after I turn out the lights is to remember what went well that day, and I review positive feelings and accomplishments from the past. This practice helps me start the next day with a positive focus.

Affirmations can be repeated throughout the day. Whenever you have a spare moment, whether at the grocery store, or stuck in traffic, imagine living your life exactly as you want. I try to give thanks for everything that I have in my life, and then focus on a goal I want to accomplish. For more information on using affirmations, I recommend reading *You Can Heal Your Life* by Louise Hay. If the sample affirmations below don't ring true for you, try using the questions I suggested for Carl.

I am creating a radiant and healthy body (imagine people complimenting you on your radiant good health).

I can love myself, as I love my neighbor (often we treat others more kindly than ourselves).

I can turn adversity into success (think about an adversity you overcame; for example, I had reading disabilities, yet graduated from college with a degree in English).

I breathe deeply, I relax completely (this can be done anywhere and anytime).

Affirmation Guidelines

- State affirmations in the positive.
- Make affirmations specific and manageable. For example, when I started thinking about writing this book, I told myself, I will write two pages a day, *not,* I will write a book.
- Make sure your affirmations are something you can control. While you can't control what other people do, you can control how you react to them.
- Involve all your senses.
- An affirmation should be something you can believe in, put your heart and soul in.
- Is the goal you're affirming realistic and achievable?

Visualize Yourself Healthy

"You get what you focus on" is an important truism for people dealing with challenging health conditions. Sights, sounds, smells, taste, and touch that we create in our mind can be useful not only for creativity, but in healing as well. When you're feeling stressed, taking time to visualize beautiful sights, sounds, and touch can provide a respite.

Many people who are sick tend to be focused on being sick. Visualization is important because if you can't imagine feeling well, you'll be less likely to actually get there. When is the last time you felt really good? What did that feel like in your body? Imagine what it would feel like to feel well, and meditate on that feeling every day, asking yourself, "What would I need to say, feel, hear, and think in order to become like my desired image?"

It's important to know that we all rely more heavily on some senses than others, and to work with your preferred sense. Most of us are some composite of visual, auditory, and kinesthetic, but it is useful to know which sense you most rely on. Because we live in a visually oriented world, most people in our culture are strongest visually. For example, when you think about a recent visit with a friend, if you see your friend's face, you might be primarily visual, while if you are more likely to remember the conversation vividly, you might have an auditory preference. Some of us are more kinesthetically inclined, and feel sensations in our body most easily. Kinesthetic people tend to be athletic. You can develop your less developed senses, for instance, by listening to music, or playing sports, or using your hands to build something.

World-class athletes "practice" by visualizing making free throws, or exploding off the block in a track meet. You can use this technique in your everyday life. For example, if you have a doctor's appointment you're nervous about, try rehearsing the visit in your mind. Imagine the visit going well. Similarly, if you are nervous about an upcoming social engagement, see yourself in the occasion, your face and body relaxed, handling the situation with new levels of ease.

Try to imagine what it will look like when you are eating healthy, taking your herbs, doing stress reduction, and exercising regularly. How will it feel to be where you want to be? Imagine looking back and seeing yourself as you are now; look back at yourself as having already made that change. How did you get there?

Begin an Exercise and Stress-Reduction Program

"Grant us the serenity to accept the things we cannot change, the courage to change the things we can, and the wisdom to know the difference." (The Serenity Prayer)

Many of us with immune disorders are worriers, and most of what we worry about is not likely to happen. A more sensible approach is to try to live "one day at a time," particularly when you are healing. In order to break the worry cycle, ask yourself, What will I do if the worst happens? The first thing to do when you feel stress is to look at it as a challenge or a learning experience. What am I learning? What is the worst that can happen? How likely is it that the worst *will* happen? Have I done everything I can realistically do? Will I remember this stress in five or ten years? How would I counsel a friend in the same situation I am in? It is also important to give yourself those things that make you feel good. The right music can help you moderate your mood, lifting you up when you're feeling down, and calming you when you are too excited. Personal favorites of mine to get going are the *William Tell Overture* and upbeat jazz music. I find classical or New Age music the most soothing when I want to relax.

Exercise & Stress Reduction

A key to healing your immune system is a commitment to one hour of exercise and stress reduction (for example, meditation, prayer, tai chi, or yoga) every day. If you don't have an hour at one time to devote to exercise and relaxation, break it up into two half-hour segments. I have seen people who make and follow through with this commitment get better, while those who cannot make this commitment often don't make a lasting improvement.

I believe that for Westerners exercise is more beneficial than relaxation techniques because it is generally easier for Westerners to quiet their mind while exercising. It's common for neophyte meditators, as soon as they sit down to meditate, to think about all the things they'd rather be doing or should be doing. When I first started to meditate, I often got shoulder and neck pains because I was too anxious about "doing it right," clearly defeating the purpose! However, meditation is a very effective method for improving health, and individuals who are able to learn and practice it correctly should do so.

Exercise increases blood flow, which then delivers oxygen more rapidly and effectively to our body tissues. Oxygen to the brain helps sharpen alertness as well as reduce anxiety and depression. Modern research has found that exercise helps the body create natural chemicals called endorphins, which help to elevate our mood. Exercise also promotes sound sleep because everything is running more efficiently.

To me, exercise means a pleasant activity done vigorously enough so that you don't spend time thinking about your problems. It's time off from your worries. As we relax, we find our personal center and become happier and healthier. On a long journey, it's important to keep the ultimate destination in mind, but it is just as important to live in the present as much as possible.

The joy is in the journey. Relaxation is essential to health, and it is even more important to relax when you are sick. You can begin to transform your body by transforming your mind. Staying present means appreciating what is around you, and not dwelling on your condition.

If possible, find a friend you can exercise with in order to give each other mutual support. The exercise you choose should be one that brings you the most enjoyment. What sports do you enjoy—aerobics, biking, rowing, jogging, hiking, racket sports, or ball games? Group exercises such as aerobics or team sports are fast-paced, so you don't have time to worry about your personal problems. Stationary bicycles, step and rowing machines, and equipment that simulates cross-country skiing are also beneficial. Swimming is said to be one of the best exercises because it puts the least amount of strain on the joints while giving you an all-around workout. If you are not in good shape, vigorous walking will do. For several reasons, walking in the country or in a park is better than walking in the city or in a shopping mall. Exposure to nature is very important to the healing process, whereas city walking exposes you to pollution as well as other discordant distractions. When walking in nature, notice how your feet feel touching the ground. Notice the flowers and animals. Notice the trees and grass. If there is a pond, notice what is reflected in it.

Some parents with toddlers buy a sports stroller with bicycle-like tires to either run or speedwalk with their young ones. When their children are older, they strap them into a child's seat on a bike. Aside from the obvious immediate benefits, youngsters are exposed to the importance of exercise at an early age, hopefully preparing them to continue with activity throughout their lives.

At the other end of the age spectrum, many of the healthiest seniors follow a program of good diet and exercise, which is why they live to such advanced ages. The YMCA I belong to offers many senior exercise activities, including aerobics and swimming, as well as outings. The only people who shouldn't follow this program are people whose doctors have told them they shouldn't walk or wheel themselves in a wheelchair, and people whose jobs involve a lot of physical work. If you fall into either of these categories, make inactivity and relaxation the greater part of your hour. A good way to end each relaxation session is self-massage (see Abdominal Self-Massage, later in this chapter).

There is no doubt that the first thirty days of making this commitment are the hardest. Keep in mind your goal of getting healthy, and focus on your mission, why it is that you want to be healthy. If necessary, get up an hour earlier. Most people find that after thirty days of practicing daily relaxation and exercise, it is their favorite part of the day, and is frequently their only time for solitude.

Abdominal Self-Massage

Abdominal self-massage can be performed daily for 10 to 20 minutes. Or it can be done anytime you feel discomfort. First warm your hands for a few minutes by shaking them, vigorously or by sitting on them. With your right hand, rub a small circle around your navel in a clockwise direction. Gradually increase the size of your circles. Experiment with different pressures. Now do

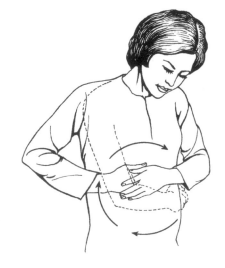

the exercise with your left hand. Finally, perform the exercise with your left hand on top of your right hand.

Tip _____

> This is a very effective exercise, but it must be practiced daily for its benefits to be felt, usually within thirty to sixty days.

Healing Effects of Prayer and Meditation

Scientific research has demonstrated the many health benefits of prayer and meditation. Studies show that prayer speeds recovery from surgery, alleviates depression, and improves the ability to handle stress. Spiritual practice has been associated with maintaining immune function under stress. Seniors who pray tend to live longer.[4] Prayer can even affect bacteria, fungi, red blood cells, and cancer cells in laboratory experiments.[5] By calming the brain, and decreasing the concentration of stress hormones circulating in our system, we can expect lower blood pressure, slower heart rate, better immune function, and less heart disease and stroke.

Dr. Herbert Benson, Harvard Medical School professor and author of the pioneering book *The Relaxation Response* in the late 1960s, conducted the early studies on the physiological effects of meditation, concluding that it decreased oxygen consumption, decreased carbon dioxide, and slowed brain waves. According to Benson, these physiological benefits last for twenty-four hours. Benson believes meditation's physiological benefits result from nitric oxide secretions interrupting the effects of norepinephrine and also causing the body to secrete endogenous opiate peptides, enkephalin, and cephalins. And all it takes to evoke that relaxation response, says Benson, is ten to twenty minutes, once or twice a day.

In a review of 1,086 scientific studies on prayer, activities such as prayer, church attendance, and the social support that comes with religious worship were found to be beneficial to health 83 percent of the time, neutral 17 percent of the time, and not harmful at all! In a study of 406 people, it was shown that prayer benefited not only the people being prayed for, but also the people doing the praying. Undirected prayer, letting go and affirming the will of a higher power and praying for "the best possible result," has been shown to yield better results than directed prayer.

Relaxation Response author Benson identified two steps that are common in meditation and prayer practices in cultures throughout the world. The first step is to repeat a word or phrase, sound, prayer, or even a repetitive movement. Then, step two, when other thoughts come to mind, disregard them and go back to the repetition. Aside from those two basic steps, whether you pray, or meditate, contemplate, or just breathe, your practice will be completely individual and unique to you. Do what makes you feel good, relaxed, connected. It doesn't have to specifically be religious, or spiritual, though it can be—bring to your practice whatever makes you feel connected to a source of support and for love, whatever that looks like to you!

Meditation is really the art of paying attention. For people with chronic immune disorders, I recommend twenty minutes of meditation in conjunction with abdominal breathing, which stimulates the lymphatic system. We were all born breathing deeply from our belly, but as we grow up, we usually come to breathe too shallowly, from the top of our lungs. Abdominal breathing is natural, and feels good once you get the hang of it. Take a deep breath, so that your stomach puffs out, filling up with air. Hold the breath for as long as you can, and as you breathe out, notice your stomach flattening on the out-breath. See how slowly you can release the breath. Try holding your stomach in for as long as possible before taking your next breath. Rather than just concentrating on the breath, it may be easier to think "breathe deeply" during the in-breath, and "relax completely" with the out-breath. Another option is to say a single word—"one," "God," "love," "release"—during the in-breath and repeating it again with the out-breath. The key to meditating is to gently steer your mind back to the breath and the repeated word. After twenty minutes of meditation, visualize yourself going about your activities with a healthy glow surrounding you, and free of your usual symptoms.

Because it doesn't provide an immediate reward, meditation is not easy for Westerners. But over time, you will notice you feel less pain, less stress, and more energy. Like any other activity, it takes time and practice to become proficient. For those who can't meditate on their own, brain wave machines can make meditation more enjoyable. Brain wave machines, also called mind machines, are devices that use light and sound to induce relaxation by altering brain waves.

Another possibility is to play progressive relaxation tapes in the background. Brain wave machines and relaxation tapes are available at bookstores, New Age stores, and some health food shops.

Take a Hot Bath

One of the most powerful weapons against the pain and anxiety associated with immune disorders is also the most gentle: a hot bath or sauna. Heat helps relax muscles and joints, and also releases stress hormones, which make it less likely that we'll overreact to stress. Ideally the bath should be as hot as you can stand. Add more hot water as necessary. Essential oils of lavender can be added. Also, herbs such as chamomile and lemon balm may be brewed as tea and added to the bath (see below for directions).

40

Some people find that a heating pad or a hot water bottle applied to painful areas works better than a bath.

Stress-Reducing Bath Number 1

Once the bath has been drawn, add 5 drops of marjoram, 5 drops of lavender, and 5 drops of chamomile. Epsom salts may then be added as well, following directions on the label. Cover up after your bath and listen to a stress-reduction tape.

Stress-Reducing Bath Number 2

Make a strong brew of chamomile and lemon balm tea, strain, and pour into the bath.

Healthy Digestion Bath

While drawing the bath, add 1 tsp. peppermint oil, or place 2 peppermint tea bags into the tub; add Epsom salts once the bath has been drawn.

Warming Bath

Pour 1–3 tsp. of powdered ginger into the bath water. If you have sensitive skin, use fresh ginger by putting a 2-inch slice in an old sock or muslin bag. You can also add 5 cinnamon sticks. You should break out into a sweat. Dry off well and cover up in a blanket as soon as you get out of the bath.

Get a Massage

You can buy a portable massager, use your own hands, or pay a massage therapist. The best alternative is a spouse or friend. I suggest beginning with the feet, and ending at the head, spending plenty of time with your stomach, spine, shoulders, neck, and forehead (see abdominal sclf-message earlier in this chapter). Mechanical self-massagers help get to hard-to-reach areas. Pressure may also be applied to tender points in the body, ears, hands, and feet to ease symptoms.

Make Time for Hobbies

"Distress causes your head to become gray; anger speeds aging; laughter makes you ten years younger." Chinese proverb

How many people work long hours and then park themselves in front of the TV? How many hours each day do you spend reading the newspaper or watching the news? Chatting on the phone? Window-shopping? None of these activities enrich your life. Many of us have forgotten simple pleasures that give the mind a rest such as hiking, walking, crafts, playing a musical instrument, or enjoying our hobbies. Success, even in small things, supports a feeling of self-confidence and self-worth. I once read about a Buddhist monk who advised his American students to give up meditation, and just spend thirty minutes a day laughing. If you must watch movies, watch comedies!

Focus on Your Goals: Have a Mission in Life

One of the most important things a sick person can have is a personal mission. For example, a friend's wife who was diagnosed with multiple sclerosis watched others who were diagnosed at the same time become confined to wheelchairs, while she had far fewer signs of her disease. Her secret? She had a mission to help kids at risk, and those children gave her purpose. Many of these children were temporarily placed in the couple's home while foster care arrangements were being made.

People who live long and well have a mission. One of the healthiest eighty-four-year-olds I know is an herbalist with whom I practice one day a week. He loves his work, and there are so many people to help, he is simply too busy to fully retire. He worked a six-day week until he turned eighty, then he began to work part time.

Healthy people cultivate positive emotions. Sick people cultivate negative emotions. Sick people often don't have faith in getting better. They surround themselves with sick people. And they don't have a strong enough reason to get well.

Act "as if" you don't have a disorder. Ask yourself what you would like to contribute. What would you like to be doing? What do you love doing? I'll bet you could take small steps toward achieving your dreams. A mission doesn't have to be something you do full time or even what you do for a living—it's a way you can live your life. Those who have overcome their conditions usually have a higher purpose to their lives that prevented them from succumbing to being victimized by their disease.

Keep a Journal

Keeping a journal is an excellent tool to help chart your progress, find inspiration, identify factors that trigger or improve symptoms, imagine creative ways to improve your health, and uncover the messages in your illness, and in your feelings about your illness.

Dedicate a page to writing down all your accomplishments and the peak experiences in your life. Read this page frequently throughout the day. Reading about your accomplishments will mobilize your subconscious to boost your immune system and reinforce the belief that you are worth healing.

Keeping a journal can also help you identify triggers. Foods, emotions, fatigue, weather, and hormones can all suppress your immune system and exacerbate symptoms. It is equally important to notice when your symptoms improve. Was there something you did to reduce stress? Did you avoid certain foods? I had a client who had chronic diarrhea, except when she traveled. As it turned out, a calcium and magnesium supplement, which she didn't take when she traveled, was causing all of her symptoms.

Ask yourself, "What do I need to change in order to have better immune health?" Don't stop until you have at least twenty ideas. Let your imagination run free. Don't edit your answers, or judge or criticize, until you've completed your list. When you've finished, go over each entry, not only focusing on the changes you can make, but also looking for hidden messages in these ideas. By the time he was near the end of his list, Bob wrote, "Move to the moon." Thinking about it, he realized that, like astronauts, he could consume liquid meals in the form of protein shakes to give him more energy.

Another excellent journaling exercise is to write a letter to those who have wronged you, or those you have wronged. You can either send the letter or simply keep it in your journal. Writing a letter to your immune disorder is also good medicine. While emotions can be explored with a counselor, therapist, or pastor, journaling is an unconventional technique that allows you to investigate hate, anger, or fear without feeling self-conscious. By writing your thoughts down, you can understand more fully some of the following issues: What is the worst possible outcome of your condition? What is the best possible outcome? What is the reason for your immune disorder? Is it because of low self-esteem? Maybe you don't feel worthy of the life you are leading. Perhaps getting a flare-up is one way to avoid aspects of your present life that you find difficult to face. Has your stress become unbearable? How could you decrease your stress level? Maybe you have never expressed, or are not aware of, how others try to control you. Is there anything your disease is trying to tell you?

For example, Cassandra named her aching gut Leo. "What are you up to now, Leo?" she would ask whenever it acted up. "What are you trying to tell me?" Another client named her insomnia Tinkerbell, and another named his fatigue Warren.

Images can also be telling. In your journal, ask yourself what images you associate with your symptoms. A very angry client got the image of a rabid pit bull. His first step in getting control over his anger was identifying when it came up. Then he could ask himself, "Why in this instance am I acting like a rabid pit bull?"

Does Your Psychology Work for You?

Roberta was a bright woman in her forties who was experiencing exhaustion, as well as muscle and joint pain. Her formal diagnosis was fibromyalgia syndrome. She thought that some of the fatigue she was experiencing was due to the drugs she was on, including narcotic pain medication and sleeping pills.

"Did you ask your doctor about going off the medication?" I asked her.

"He said that would be a bad idea."

"Did he say why?"

She shrugged. "He said I would probably have to be on it for several years because people with my condition don't improve quickly."

I gave her several examples of people who had come into our clinic who recovered 50 percent or more of their energy within a few months. I said that in order to heal and regain her strength she might have to see another doctor who was more supportive of her getting off her drugs, or choosing alternate drugs that would be less sedating.

"Oh, I can't do that," Roberta protested. "I like my doctor. He's a nice man. I just feel so bad, though, when I need two or three naps just to make it through the day."

"Healing almost always requires an examination of our habitual thoughts, beliefs, and behavior," I told her. "To feel like our old selves again, we usually need to change some of these habits, to become our new selves. Ask yourself if your thoughts, beliefs, and actions are strengthening or weakening you. Would finding a doctor who could help you reevaluate your medication be strengthening or weakening?"

"It would make me stronger."

"Good, so that's one thing you need to do. Does taking two or three naps a day make you stronger or weaker?"

"It makes me stronger."

"Good. There's nothing wrong with taking a brief nap during the day to recharge your batteries."

"I'm worried about my caffeine consumption."

"Does worrying about how much caffeine you're consuming make you stronger or weaker?"

"It makes me feel bad because without the caffeine I feel like I'd never be able to make it out of the house. But my friend Rosemary said that caffeine isn't good for people with chronic fatigue and sleep problems."

"If you want to get better you are going to have to make priorities. Once again, will quitting caffeine make you stronger or weaker?"

"It would make me weaker, at least at first."

"Then quit later." We proceeded with this exercise for the next twenty minutes. When her appointment was over, Roberta had a plan of action and a new way to prioritize her life.

Confession and Forgiveness Are Good for the Body and Soul
Forgiveness and Letting Go

Many people believe that seeking outside help is a sign of weakness, so they tend to isolate themselves, which only adds to their anger and depression. Actually, it takes strength to realize that you need help. Share your suffering with a friend, counselor, or minister. Realizing that you are not alone in your suffering is often helpful. Chances are in this world with six billion people on it, there are thousands if not millions going through exactly what you are going through at this moment. Telling someone about our worries can help us gain perspective on them.

Your primary worry may not be your immune disorder; it may be work or a family conflict. Relationships can be a source of stress, frequently because we enter into a relationship with unrealistic expectations. These expectations are heightened by the often unreal, romantic views of relationships presented to us through films, television, and magazines. Relationship transitions—such as marriage, divorce, childbirth, sickness, and death—all must be discussed and resolved. A counselor does not solve problems, but helps people understand their problems, communicate their needs, work out compromises, and develop coping skills.

We often keep our worries and troubles to ourselves, which usually just makes them loom larger. It takes a tremendous amount of energy to have a secret, energy that could be used for healing. It takes energy to be constantly on guard about everything you say and do so that nobody will find out. Your secret may be your immune disorder, the fact that you were raped, were abused, can't read, can't do math, have an addiction, had a teen pregnancy, or are gay.

Dr. Howard Liebgold is a well-known physician who, after conquering his own phobia, is now devoted to teaching other people how to cure theirs. "My secret was my claustrophobia," says Liebgold. "I was terrified that if anyone found out that a doctor, a specialist, and chief of a department was less than perfect, I would be ridiculed and probably fired. . . . Years later when I revealed my 'terrible secret' in an article to two million Kaiser members—I got a raise. . . . Every time I told another person about my phobia, I desensitized myself."

Although you can't change the past, you can accept, forgive, and move on. "When you are able to share your secret with your universe, you'll have taken the first step to dealing with the pain and burden of carrying that secret. As I did, you'll soon find out that you can handle it."[6]

What secrets do you have? Could you tell them to a counselor, priest, minister, or friend? Even just writing your secret in a journal is a way to be good to your immune system, if you feel like you aren't ready to tell anyone.

"If we get stuck in resentment and anger, we can build toxins inside ourselves and cling to them in a way that harms us. Healing is the answer. See the past for what it is, then forgive and let go. This is the way to find peace."[7] Lingering resentments, anger, or bitterness can hamper healing. As Mother Teresa said, "If we really want to love, we must learn how to forgive." Ask yourself if you really want to continue to be angry, resentful, or bitter. If the answer is no, the best thing you can do is to forgive the person or situation that is the focus of your bad feelings. When you forgive, you no longer need to be a victim. When you forgive, you do it for yourself—not for the good of the other people involved. You can forgive yourself, your ex, and your family members as a way to make peace with yourself.

Forgiveness does not mean what the other person did was okay. It means that you need to live with that person, or work for them. Forgiveness does not mean you've forgotten what happened. If we get into the car with a drunk driver, and they get us into an accident, we can forgive them, but we don't ever have to get into the car with them again. You can forgive your ex-spouse without having to live with them, or be friends with them.

Don't wait until the other parties have apologized—they may never apologize. Forgive when you are tired of carrying all that ill will around with you. Forgiveness is not surrender, but a decision *not* to be stuck in resentment.

When you forgive someone, you'll probably notice that you feel better immediately, only to feel the old resentments come up again later. If this happens, and it probably will, you'll need to forgive them again. Forgiving is usually not a one-shot deal. We can hate the person for what they did, what they stand for, but we can never change what they did. We can only change what the experience means to us. It's easiest to be honest and admit it to yourself. "Fred hurt me, and I will probably always hate him for it, but I can try to make sure something like this never happens again, and I can forgive him because it's better for me."

As a young man, Arnold was raped in a New York City subway. He never reported the attack. Even after moving to California, taking antidepressants, and seeing a therapist, he would sometimes wake up at 3 a.m. dripping with sweat, having thrown the covers off the bed, red hot with rage. When Arnold's therapist first suggested he forgive his attacker, he almost walked out of the session. The therapist then clarified that he was suggesting Arnold forgive the attacker for Arnold's own good. The therapist pointed out that the attacker had probably been abused in a similar way and would, eventually, probably be caught and imprisoned. The therapist encouraged Arnold to try to avoid thinking about the attack, and when he did think about it, to watch his thoughts as if they were on a movie screen in fast forward and rapid rewind, repeating "I forgive you because that will be best for me". Arnold did this exercise in the therapist's office, and repeated the exercise at home when he had memories of the experience.

Get Support

The old adage "Misery loves company" has some truth—with a twist. Many patients want someone to really care about how they feel. In the movie *Wit,* actress Emma Thompson plays a patient with advanced ovarian cancer, in a teaching hospital. Physicians and hospital staff are continually asking how she is, but only one nurse takes enough time to look at her in a kind way and sit with her. One of the reasons the patient in *Wit* goes downhill so quickly is that she is prescribed a deadly dosage of chemotherapy. Another reason we see her go downhill so quickly is that she has no support from friends or family.

In addition to asking for the kind of support you want from friends and family, you can join a formal support group for extra help. Dr. David Spiegel and his associates at Stanford Medical School[8] have documented that patients with metastatic breast cancer who attended a weekly support group had significantly better health than, and lived twice as long as, those who did not attend the weekly support group. In addition, those in the support group had less anxiety, confusion, fatigue, and mood disturbance. In another study, published in the *Archives of General Psychiatry,*[9] among sixty-eight patients with malignant melanoma, those attending six weekly support groups were found to have better NK cell activity, improved mood, and a longer life span.

According to Dr. Spiegel, the benefits of support groups include[10] receiving encouragement to eat well, exercise regularly, and get plenty of sleep. He also suggests that support groups may help improve immune functioning, reduce stress, and promote better communications with health professionals.

What to look for in a group? Find a group that is specific to your condition so that you can share with people who have challenges similar to your own. You should feel understood and comforted by people in the group. If you don't feel comfortable with the first group you try, find another group. There may be self-help groups, or groups led by professionals.

Friends and family can be very helpful. In *Wit,* the main character has no friends or family visiting her until the end. When people visit and bring cards and flowers, you are reminded that people care about you, that you have a life aside from your illness. Feeling loved, wanted, and needed gives you a reason to get better.

It's even more empowering to ask for exactly the kind of help that you want. People are often embarrassed or shy about offering help, or they're at a loss and just don't know what to do. They'll likely be delighted if you make a list of things you could use help with. It may be preparing a meal, driving you to an appointment, or going to the library to bring you books. Communicate what you are looking for clearly to your friends and family. Maybe you want somebody who will just listen to you without judgment or trying to "fix it." Whereas one person may want understanding, another person may want to hear solutions. When Paula's mother visited her, she would always try to change the subject away from Paula's condition. At least you're not in India starving, she'd tell Paula, or at least you're not dying, at least you don't have to go to work, and you have a supportive husband. "Mom, I just don't want to hear about all the starving children in India right now," Paula would say. Once Paula's mother realized that Paula wanted someone to just listen, she stopped changing the subject, and just listened to what Paula had to say.

It's also completely okay to end discussions that are painful or overwhelming to you. For instance, John's partner Jerry continually wanted to discuss treatment options based on research he had done on the Internet. After an hour, John had to just say, "Thank you for doing all this work. I just can't deal with it right now. Let's find another time." The result is that Jerry felt validated for doing the research, and was fine with shelving the conversation until John felt more up for it.

"You've just lost your boob and your hair. It doesn't mean you're not feminine," is not what Collette wanted to hear from her husband. What she wanted to hear was, "It's not important to me that you lost your breast and hair. I still love you."

The Importance of Conserving Your Energy

It's important to have ample energy in order to maximize our immune health. In addition to doing strengthening practices like tai chi and qi gong, it's important not to stretch yourself too thin. If you want to maximize your immune health, it helps to think of your health as a savings account where you make deposits, but seldom make withdrawals. You can make deposits by reducing your daily stress, by increasing your daily exercise, by taking herbs and other nutritional supplements, and by learning to take one day at a time and say "no" to excess commitments. In other words, don't push yourself beyond your abilities.

For example, when Rob was trying to cope with his mother's lung cancer and a close friend who was dying of AIDS, his boss needed time off and placed Rob in charge of running the company. For almost six months, Rob battled one cold and flu after another, cold sores, and finally came down with mononucleosis, for which he was bedridden for several weeks. Although he was a great son and friend, taking over the company was more than his immune and nervous systems could stand.

It has been my observation that many people with immune disorders are unduly influenced by other people. It's good to be concerned for other people, but some people overdo it to their detriment. An irritable bowel syndrome client named Ellen comes to mind. She is a nurse and mother, who was on several civic committees. Her problem was not being able to say no. "They're running me ragged!" she told me one day. I referred her to a self-help book, *The Feeling Good Handbook* by Dr. David Burns, and asked her if she could feel the consequences of people's demands. She replied, "When they ask me for something, I can feel my stomach tightening up." I told her that whenever she felt that uncomfortable feeling to visualize "pulling a plug" out of her stomach to unplug from the feeling. You might also want to try crossing your arms over your abdomen for protection.

One of the paradoxes we see in our clinic is that when we help someone regain their strength and vitality, they immediately want to go out and spend it all at once. For example, Mary came to our clinic complaining of fatigue. She woke up tired after twelve hours of sleep, and unless she took at least one nap during the day, she couldn't function. She also got frequent infections, including a cold or flu every month or so.

After taking the herbs and nutritional supplements we recommended for two weeks, Mary's energy improved. Even though she hadn't been able to take her kids to the shopping mall in two years, the first thing she did when she felt her energy return was go to the shopping mall. She did fine in the first store she went in, but in the second store she began to wonder if she was going to be able to drive home. Her third stop was her last. She got dizzy in the store, and had to sit down in the nearest chair she could find. The store manager called Mary's sister, who came

53

and brought her home. After three days of lying in bed, Mary was back to where she'd been before taking the herbs, all because she did too much too soon.

In Mary's mind, she should be able to drive and visit stores in the shopping mall because she used to work eight- to twelve-hour days and then shop for the whole family. But that wasn't the Mary that came to our clinic. That was the old Mary. We acknowledged Mary for making the effort to drive to the shopping mall and visit a few stores, and suggested that the next time when she went to the mall, she use her fatigue as a signal to either rest in her car or start making the trip back. We also suggested that she not compare herself to her old self, but focus on how far she had come in just two weeks on the herbs.

"I felt like such a failure," Mary said in our office, fighting off tears.

"Why?" I asked her. "You hadn't been to the shopping mall in two years. That's a major accomplishment!"

"I didn't used to be a basket case. I used to have a regular life," she said.

By resting for three days, Mary allowed her batteries to recharge. Once a person's batteries are recharged, the person is stronger not only physically, but also mentally, emotionally, and spiritually. Mary left the clinic feeling better. Over the next three months, she built her energy by taking herbs, enrolling in a local yoga class, trying to walk every day, and trying to eat protein with each meal.

"I felt like I could have driven to the shopping mall, but I took your advice and conserved my energy," Mary told me at her next appointment. "It wasn't an emergency that I go shopping." The next time she went to the mall, Mary went to one store and left before she was exhausted.

An underlying principle of Chinese medicine is that everything is always changing, like the seasons. Accepting the changes, and adapting to them, can greatly lighten our load. I told Mary that in many Asian traditions, life is seen as unfolding in cycles of seven years. Just because a person is sick for a few years, does not mean they will be that way for the rest of their life.

Ask Your Body

Our body is always communicating with us. Unfortunately, we are often not listening. Our body can't talk to us in words, but it lets us know when it's happy, and it lets us know when something is wrong by discomfort sensations.

Use the meditation exercise (see Healing Effects of Prayer and Meditation, earlier in this chapter) for a few minutes to calm your mind. You should do this exercise in an environment free from any distractions.

Place your hands over your heart and navel, and ask, Is there anything you would like to tell me? Become aware of any sensation. You may hear an inner voice. You may get an image, or you may have a certain feeling in your body. Perhaps there's a smell, or a taste in your mouth. Ask your body, What is this sensation telling me? Are there actions I need to take that are different? Are there things I can do to help my immune system? If you are not sure what these sensations mean, ask yourself, "Even though I don't know what these images, voices, or sensations mean, if I did know, what would they mean?"

Kevin got an image of something vague chasing him. For several days, he asked himself what the image meant. While reading about imaging and visualization, he had an insight that, rather than his immune system eating Kevin up, he could turn the tables, and turn around and chase what had been chasing him. He found out that as he visualized changing direction, the fear began to lift. As he ran toward what had been chasing him, it changed direction, and started shrinking, smaller and smaller. The faster he ran, the smaller it shrank, until it was the size of a tiny microbe that he could overtake. For Kevin, this simple change signaled a turnaround in his health.

Balance Your Hormones
Balance Your Yin and Yang

The endocrine glands—which include the hypothalamus, pituitary, thyroid, and adrenal glands—release hormones that influence every part of the body. Hormones regulate metabolism, mood, growth and development, and sexual function. Disorders of the thyroid and adrenal glands, in particular, can mimic immune disorders.

In Chinese medicine terms, the kidney controls the endocrine system. The kidney system is in charge of generating and storing Qi, or vital energy. If your kidney qi is strong, you will be able to think clearly, decisively, and with courage. Deficient kidney qi is associated with fear. The kidneys are considered the mother organ—they support all the other organs. If, for example, the liver gets tapped out due to stress, anger, or rage, the body must draw added support from the kidneys.

The endocrine system, in Chinese medicine, balances yin and yang in the body. Yang is related to the reactive sympathetic nervous system, which revs your body up when you're under stress. Yang speeds up the metabolism and releases energy. Yang is warming and transformative. Yin, on the other hand, is related to the parasympathetic nervous system, which is at work when we are relaxed. Yin stores energy and slows the metabolism, is cooling, soothing, and maintaining. Kidney yang seems related to epinephrine and norepinephrine secreted by the adrenal medulla, as well as some pituitary and thyroid hormones. Kidney yin relates to the adrenal cortex's secretion of cortisol.[11]

Thyroid Gland. The thyroid is a butterfly-shaped gland located on the neck, just under the Adam's apple. The thyroid makes hormones that regulate metabolism and organs, and when it's not working properly, it can cause problems throughout the body. Signs of hypothyroidism—an underactive thyroid that's not making enough thyroid hormone—include fatigue, weight gain, mood swings, forgetfulness, hoarse voice, dry, coarse skin and hair, trouble swallowing, feeling cold, increased cholesterol, heavy or irregular periods or trouble getting pregnant, and an enlarged thyroid. At the other end of the spectrum, hyperthyroidism—an overactive thyroid secreting excess thyroid hormone—may cause weight loss, heat, irritability, nervousness, muscle weakness and tremors, irregular menstrual periods, disturbed sleep, eye irritations, heart palpitations, frequent or loose bowel movements, and an enlarged thyroid. Whether it's overactive or underactive, a disorder of the thyroid can be diagnosed with a blood test measuring thyroid stimulating hormone, or TSH.[12]

Adrenal Glands. Located at the top of each kidney, the adrenal glands play a significant role in the body's ability to adapt to stress, whether emotional stress, or physical stress such as injury, infection, or allergic reaction. The adrenal glands produce the hormone cortisol (also called hydrocortisone), which helps the body maintain homeostasis under stress, and counteracts allergic and inflammatory reactions. In low concentrations, cortisol supports the immune system. It helps the body make antibodies; for example, the body makes more cortisol in the early stages of an infection. In high doses, however, cortisol suppresses the immune system. Over time, excessive cortisol can promote aging, loss of bone density, and heart disease.

The hormones secreted by the adrenal glands are called corticosteroids. Synthetic derivatives of corticosteroids like prednisone are useful for treating immune conditions, but long-term use of these drugs decreases the adrenal cortex's ability to produce cortisol, leading to adrenal insufficiency. Symptoms of adrenal insufficiency include fatigue, especially under stress, low blood sugar, sugar cravings, dizziness, fatigue, brain fog, poor concentration, poor coping ability, depression, weight loss, headaches, allergies, asthma, reduced libido, insomnia, and certain autoimmune conditions. Stress, chemicals in the environment, and the excessive use of pharmaceutical and recreational drugs can lead to adrenal insufficiency and burnout.

Severe adrenal burnout symptoms include low blood pressure, hypoglycemia, weight loss, digestive symptoms, and joint and muscle aches, and may be diagnosed as Addison's disease. Treatment may include oral steroids, typically administered along with salt. Acute adrenal failure is a medical emergency that requires hospitalization. Typically the patient becomes dehydrated due to diarrhea and vomiting, and may go into shock or lose consciousness. Increased protein intake, B vitamins, and meditation can help improve the adrenal function, over time. Also, adaptogenic herbs and kidney tonic herbs can be administered by a trained practitioner to address adrenal symptoms.

Natural Methods for Reducing Inflammation

The purpose of inflammation is to protect us from infection and promote wound healing. Chronic inflammation may begin at one site, but then spread throughout the body and attack other areas. Chronic inflammatory disorders include arthritis, allergies, asthma, and cardiovascular disease. Aspirin and ibuprofen (Motrin, Advil), Naproxen sodium (Aleve), and Celebrex are examples of popular anti-inflammatory drugs. Chronic inflammation is caused or exacerbated by a variety of factors, including:

- Certain foods promote inflammation, especially sweets, deep-fried foods, and foods you are allergic to.
- Inhaled allergens, such as pollen and mold, also cause inflammation.
- Being overweight increases the body's production of inflammation-causing substances.
- Physical injuries can produce chronic inflammation, especially if they don't heal properly or are repeated.
- Infections such as chronic colds and flus, hepatitis, HIV, parasites, and yeast (candida) overgrowth contribute to inflammation.
- Sunburn, pollution, and smoking also promote inflammation.

Healthy habits can keep inflammation at bay. Fish oil, antioxidant vitamins, and many herbs can be used to reduce inflammation. A diet rich in fruits and vegetables provides vitamin C, carotenoids, and flavonoids, which reduce inflammation. Olive oil also has anti-inflammatory properties. Finally, I've observed that clients engaged in a daily stress-reduction program have less incidence of inflammatory disease.

Challenge Your Limiting Beliefs

"Belief is a powerful healing agent. Simply by opening our minds, we may be surprised by our own inner strength."[13] According to the dictionary, beliefs are the mental acceptance of the truth. There are some strange beliefs out there. For example, some people believe that men never visited the moon; it was all done with mirrors. On a remote island, it is believed that the best way to raise children is by having the aunt, not the mother, raise the children.

I'll bet that many of your beliefs about yourself are equally strange. What are some of the beliefs that you had at one time that you no longer believe? Perhaps when you were young you believed, "I'll never learn how to ride a bike," or "I'll never learn to swim," yet soon after, you were riding a bike and swimming. Another way of looking at negative beliefs is that they're like computer software with a bug. If you got a file with a virus, wouldn't you clean it out, and install a new program?

What are some of the negative beliefs you have about yourself and your health? Do you ever think things like, *I'll never heal. I'll die a horrible death. I never do anything right.*

Because beliefs are mental, they are subject to change at any time. In fact, they are changing, constantly. If you've ever tried meditating, you've experienced this phenomenon.

Challenge your limiting beliefs. Look at the evidence. What ideas do you have that bother you? Please list three negative beliefs you have about yourself here:

1. _____

2. _____

3. _____

What evidence do you have that these beliefs are true? More importantly, does your negative belief serve you well, or does it undermine your health and well-being?

Many people define their health on the basis of genetics. "My dad died from a heart attack at age forty." "Cancer runs in my family." "I have alcoholic genes."

One problem with these beliefs is that they are disempowering and can lead to self-fulfilling prophecies. Although you may have an alcoholic mother or father, you probably also have close relatives who are not alcoholics. Who didn't die an early death? Who got sick, and then got better, and is now healthier than ever before? I've met many people who were never healthier than after they had their first stroke, or after they were diagnosed with HIV or hepatitis, or even cancer.

Pretend you are a detective on your favorite detective show (mine is *Columbo*), and investigate your beliefs. Have you always had these beliefs, or are they new? Do you have these beliefs only when you are in a bad mood, or tired, or when you feel bad? For example, if your belief is "I never do anything right," that's not true because you made the right decision by reading this book and learning about how to support your immune health. If you believe you'll die a horrible death, even if that belief were to prove true, how does it help you to dwell on this unpleasant possibility? Notice how you feel when you think these negative thoughts—do they give you a headache, make you feel anxious? And when you think positive thoughts, notice how the tension in your body drops away, a peaceful feeling settles over you, a smile comes to your lips. How would you rather feel?

Negative beliefs can also come to us in the labels used by people around us, such as cancer patients, AIDS victims, and crack baby. One of my clients was told, "Your vision will not improve. You will always be legally blind." It turned out that Mike had a condition called diabetic retinopathy. Mike got a second opinion, and a few months after adjusting his diabetes medications and taking special eye herbs and nutrients, he was able to read headlines and large print. Six months later, he was no longer legally blind.

Each day in our clinic, we meet people who are given various sentences by their physicians. Physicians may do this because they are uncaring, or because they truly believe that it is best to not give false hopes. But it is important not to buy into the negative beliefs of others. Willy came to our clinic because he was supposed to die in six months of liver cancer. Two years later he is still going strong. One of the reasons he's still going strong is that he wasn't afraid to challenge his doctor's negative beliefs. Willy decided he would show his doctor by getting healthy.

Healthy people have cancer, too—it's just controlled by the immune system. Do you find you often exaggerate symptoms? If you find you say things like, "My head is killing me," this is a negative belief that can be challenged. When was the last time a headache killed anybody? Try adding the word "healing" next time you catch yourself complaining about a symptom. "I am healing my cold. I am healing my chronic fatigue."

See if you can install some positive beliefs. What do you do well? Who loves you? What do you feel strongly about? What are positive beliefs that others have shared about you, even if you do not fully believe them? Can you act "as if" you had stronger, more self-supporting beliefs?

If you had more positive beliefs, what would they be?

_____

_____

_____

_____

Simply by reviewing your list of positive thoughts every day, you will be moving away from attacking yourself and your immune system, and moving in the direction of supporting yourself.

Question Your Diagnosis

If you have recently received a serious diagnosis, it makes sense to get a second opinion. Doctors, as well as laboratories, make mistakes. The possibility of error is a part of any diagnosis. Research at Johns Hopkins University has show that 1.4 percent of the time pathologists make diagnostic mistakes and sometimes wrongly diagnose cancer. In prostate cancer, mistakes are made 20 percent of the time, in determining the stage of cancer. Conditions such as heart disease, diabetes, and arthritis can trigger false positives in some tests. This can result in wrong treatments being used.[14]

A diagnosis can be devastating, particularly when your doctor tells you you're going to die soon. We may be relieved that our condition is finally labeled, but then sink into despair. At first we were miserable because things were so unclear, but now some nasty things are all too clear. We are suddenly confronted with a morass of technical information on our condition and possible treatments. We have decisions to make. Remember that your diagnosis is just a way of categorizing your symptoms to identify the best possible treatment. While doctors may define us by our symptoms, we don't have to define ourselves that way.

Beliefs guide our actions and thoughts. The placebo response demonstrates that we can heal ourselves if we believe in the potency of the medicine. How healthy do you believe you are? Studies have shown that people who believed that they were in poor health, were three times more likely to die in the subsequent seven years than those who believed they were in good health.[15] Up to 30 percent of heart attack patients never fully recover because they believe they will never fully recover, and so they fail to adopt healthy new behaviors that would support their recovery. In contrast, patients who have a positive vision and goals adopt healthy dietary and exercise habits because they can see beyond their illness.

Don't become your diagnosis, as Beth did. Beth complained of muscle pain, and after a battery of tests was diagnosed with fibromyalgia. Beth attended a support group, where she found out she could receive disability assistance for her condition. A year later, she was unable to work and had lost track of her old friends. The only people she associated with were from her fibromyalgia support group. She no longer gardened or walked because that's not what people with fibromyalgia do. She took great interest in all her symptoms, because her new friends liked to talk about their symptoms. She ate special pain-control diets, read constantly about her illness, deposited her disability checks, and quickly became one of my most disabled fibromyalgia clients. Beth became her diagnosis. Do you handicap yourself by medicalizing yourself, identifying with your illness, losing sight of your unique individuality? By not identifying your self with your illness you may wriggle your way out of its grasp. Beth is an example of someone who didn't question her diagnosis or her well-meaning friends.

If a diagnosis can be devastating, a prognosis can literally be deadly. When Maude's oncologist told her she had six months to live, he probably didn't explain that, as with any prognosis, he wasn't really talking about her, that his prognosis was one doctor's view that a hypothetical average patient with Maude's type of cancer would die in six months. Without knowing a great deal about Maude as a person, it would be impossible for anyone to make a decent prognosis. Far more than lab values go into making a person. A person is made up of their experiences, their habits, their support system, and their beliefs. Unfortunately, Maude believed her oncologist, and she died within six months, just as he had predicted.

On the other hand, when another oncologist told Bertram he had six months to live, he cursed the doctor out. "You have no business telling me that!" was his response. Bertram quickly found an oncology practice that supported his desire to try natural methods, and assured him that they would not "give him a sentence." Bertram is alive today. Although Bertram's recovery was based on many things—his zest for life, the natural therapies he used, a different drug protocol—one thing for certain is that he did not share Maude's belief that the "doctor is always right."

Telling Stories

Our beliefs are the stories we tell ourselves about how the world works. With chronic illness, the story usually begins with symptoms that don't go away. As with any story, there are many viewpoints to explore. Stories typically involve conflict and a leading character. The conflict may be external—for example, a foreign microbe or germ that multiplies in your immune system when it's weak—or internal, as in autoimmune disease, when the body attacks itself. Can you rewrite your story from the perspective of a survivor?

Jeremy rewrote his story. When Jeremy was first diagnosed with advanced liver disease due to hepatitis, his doctor told him it was too late for any treatment, and that he had a year to live. After spending a few weeks feeling blue, he called up his daughter-in-law, who was a natural healer. She suggested he come into our clinic for herbal treatment.

I told Jeremy that it may be true that the "average" person with his diagnosis would be dead within a year, but that people with the same diagnosis have lived ten years or longer. While the "average" person accepts their diagnosis, survivors get second opinions and investigate natural healing options. I suggested that Jeremy see another specialist to get a second opinion. I also made a number of lifestyle and dietary suggestions, including taking herbs to regenerate liver function. One year later, Jeremy had lost a considerable amount of weight, had more energy than before his terminal diagnosis, and had just gotten back from an enjoyable vacation. His new doctor said his condition has improved so much they may try a new experimental procedure.

Looking forward five years, what steps will you need to take to be healthy and happy? Run a movie of yourself in five years, happy, healthy, and able to achieve the goals you have set for yourself. What would that look like?

If five years seems like too much, try looking one year ahead. After her cancer diagnosis, Sandy's goal was to make it to her 50th wedding anniversary. She ran a movie in her mind. Sandy was healthy and able to enjoy the event, eating her favorite cake, having a hundred people toast her and her husband. She had no trouble seeing this image vividly, as well as hearing people congratulating her. She could step into the wonderful feeling, tasting the cake and smelling the roses on the table. As she rehearsed this future movie over and over, her mind was formulating a plan. She would need to follow both her doctors' instructions, as well as try vitamins, herbs, and hypnosis. When it came time for her actual golden anniversary party, everybody remarked that Sandy looked better than she had in years.

Cope with Pain

Jon Kabat-Zinn, Ph.D., author of the highly recommended book, *Wherever You Go, There You Are,*[16] pioneered the use of meditation to help patients with chronic pain at the University of Massachusetts Medical Center. Studies have shown that meditating by paying attention to the pain and the various sensations in your body is more effective than trying to tune out the pain. There are many pathways in the brain and the central nervous system that can modify the perception of pain, and through meditation, patients can actually teach themselves to feel less pain.

Explore new ways of controlling your pain, such as acupuncture, hypnosis, or imagery. Prepare yourself for setbacks—they are only temporary and happen to everyone. In his book *Mastering Pain: A Twelve Step Program for Coping with Chronic Pain,* Dr. Richard Sternbach,[17] director of the Pain Treatment Center in San Diego, makes the following suggestions for coping with chronic pain:

1. Accept your pain.
2. Use work, hobbies, and recreation to distract yourself from your pain.
3. Take medications, herbs, and supplements as prescribed.
4. Get fit and stay fit.
5. Use relaxation techniques.
6. Keep active.
7. Pace yourself.
8. Ask for help from family and friends.
9. Be open and honest with your health professionals.
10. Stay hopeful.

Tracking your level of discomfort in a journal is one way to become more curious about your condition. Can you describe the sensations you are afraid of? Can you ask the discomfort what it is trying to show you? Notice exactly where the discomfort is located. Does it take up a lot of space? Or is it a tiny pinprick? Gauge its intensity. How does it feel? Is it a spasm or rigid, burning or ice-cold, stabbing or throbbing? If you close your eyes and tune into the sensation, can you notice it shift in intensity or location? If the sensation were a color, what color would it be? If you listen very closely, is there a sound or voice associated with the discomfort? Can you change this voice? When Gloria first tuned into her sensations, she could hear a horrible, agonized *ahhhhh* sound. By imagining the *ahhhhh* sound to be a throaty sign of ecstasy, she took the bite out of her pain immediately! You may also be able to picture a sensation, and experiment with changing its color. For example, Vic saw his wrist pain as being red and black. When he visualized a soothing ocean blue color in his wrist, the discomfort vanished.

Experiment with moving your body more. Walking, swimming, yoga, and tai chi are all gentle ways to get your body moving. Sometimes you need to push past some initial discomfort in order to conquer the pain. Champion athletes frequently have pain. Many of my clients who are top-caliber bicyclists actually enjoy pushing past the pain. **Something in their psychology tells them pain is good, and makes them feel alive.** Of course, you should always see a health care professional to make sure you are not injuring a joint or a muscle, but magic doesn't happen without pushing through some discomfort.

See a holistic health professional who can advise you on the use of herbs and nutritional supplements. When taken correctly, herbs and supplements can reduce your level of pain, and reduce your reliance on pharmaceutical medications. While the appropriate use of drugs is sometimes warranted, often people use these medications to chase symptoms, and the underlying cause of their pain is not discovered, causing a vicious cycle of stronger and stronger drugs, with more debilitating side effects.

Power of Music

*"This little light of mine
I'm going to let it shine
Let it shine, let it shine, let it shine."* [18]

One of the most self-affirming things you can do is to sing and play inspirational songs. Many of us are self-conscious about the way we sound, so we don't sing. Many people sing to themselves in the shower, but you can also sing to yourself in the car, out in nature, or practically anytime you are alone.

There are several aspects of music that can be healing. First, there is the melody, or the particular way a song is structured, along with the compositional parts such as which instruments are used.

Then there is the rhythm. In Africa, drumming can have many meanings. Drumming is used to celebrate, to communicate, and even to heal. And vigorous drumming releases tension.

Lyrics can also heal directly, or transport us back to a special moment.

Of course, you can listen to music purely for enjoyment, and this also probably has a beneficial effect on the immune system.

There are many ways you can make music work for you. For example, if you are blue or sad, listen to uplifting music to help change your mood.

Singing is energizing! I use music that has a strong beat to motivate me while I am driving to the gym, or to any activity I find challenging.

When you are humming a tune, you emphasize particular uplifting lyrics, or create your own. That's right; simply borrow the tune of your favorite song and put any lyric you want to the tune. If possible, say the words out loud. By singing positive lyrics out loud, whether or not you have created them, you fully engage your nervous system. You can have even more fun by imitating the delivery of your favorite singer. The key is to lose yourself in the music or lyrics. If you can't picture the passion of your favorite singer in a live performance, watch them on video. Notice the gestures they use, the facial expressions, the way they breathe and move their body. How do they build emotional intensity? Why not use these elements to push you into peak immune performance?

Food Tips
Digestive Healing

Immune Eating Plan
1. Always eat breakfast
2. Make sure to get adequate protein, at least .5 g. of protein for every pound that you weigh*
3. Enjoy fresh fruits and vegetables
4. Investigate alternative grains such as rice, buckwheat, millet and quinoa

5. Identify food triggers: avoid foods your body does not like
6. Stay away from raw fish and undercooked meats and eggs
7. Limit sweets including artificial sweeteners like fructose
8. Use high-quality oils, such as extra virgin olive oil. Use flax, walnut, or sesame oil as a garnish
9. Drink at least 64 oz. of pure water per day
10. Enjoy your food

*Certain individuals, particularly those with liver and kidney problems, may need less protein.

Eat Immune-Enhancing Foods

A diet rich in a wide variety of fresh fruits and vegetables is the cornerstone of an immune-friendly diet. By eating at least five half-cup servings each of fruits and vegetables, you can get a wide spectrum of nutrient-rich phytochemicals that support the elimination of wastes from the body. In addition, filling up on good-for-you foods decreases cravings for junk foods such as excessive sweets and fats that tend to curb immune response. Because so many people are allergic to it, it's best to avoid wheat, but eating healthy grains such as rice, millet, buckwheat, and quinoa promotes good digestive function and also reduces food cravings.

Adequate protein is also essential for proper immune function. A few ounces of protein with every meal support energy levels. Fish like salmon, and game meats like rabbit and venison, all contain healthy omega-3 oils, which support a healthy immune response. Other meats and poultry, particularly red meats, contain blood-building components.

Breakfasts to support the immune system include eggs and protein shakes. If you don't have soy intolerance, soy protein powders are also good. A shake with rice, soy or pea protein powder, plenty of fruit, and hot grain cereal makes a delicious and nutritious breakfast.

For lunch and dinner, cooked vegetables and a small amount of grain and protein are excellent. Although salads may be contraindicated if you have digestive disorders, they can provide an additional source of nutrient-rich vegetables. Fruits can be eaten between meals as snacks. Be sure to use olive oil for cooking, in place of oils that promote oxidation like corn or soy oils. Healthy oils that are heat-sensitive, and therefore not suitable for cooking, include sesame, flax, and walnut oils.

Foods to specifically avoid are excessive sweets, breads, wheat, dairy products, fatty foods, coffee, alcoholic beverages, and soda. Many of these foods contain allergens, which increase oxidation and put a burden on the immune system. (See the section on Allergies in Chapter Three, "Conditions and Treatments.") From a Chinese medicine perspective, many of these ingredients cause excess heat.

To eat an immune-healthy diet, we need to consume moderate to high levels of protein, vegetables, fruits, and healthy oils and to minimize the use of unhealthy fats, sweets, artificial sweeteners, dyes, and additives. The immune system depends on adequate nutrition, and unless you can adequately digest and absorb the food you eat, it's likely that your health will be less than optimal. While a health professional can come up with an individual eating plan for you, here are some general guidelines for people with an active immune disorder.

- An easy way to immediately improve your digestion is to eat more slowly, and chew your food well, at least seven times before swallowing. Digestion actually begins in the mouth. By chewing well, we are mixing food with saliva, which is rich in digestive enzymes. Eating slowly improves the digestive process by allowing your body to concentrate on digesting. It is theorized that many Europeans have healthier hearts than Americans because they spend more time eating. When we eat on the go, or skip meals, we send "fight-or-flight" signals to our body that don't allow the proper assimilation of food.

◆ Eating smaller, more frequent meals is a digestive-friendly habit. Many Americans overwhelm their digestive systems by depriving themselves at breakfast, eating lunch on the run, and then overburdening their digestive tracts with a "hearty" dinner. Try eating four to six light meals per day, instead of that one bigger meal. You'll most likely feel more satisfied and less stressed, and it will be easier for your body to receive everything you are giving it.

◆ Try to eat as many colorful fruits and vegetables as possible, the more color the better.

◆ If you have fatigue, digestive symptoms, or joint pain, we suggest a digestive clearing diet (see Chapter Four).

◆ If you are sensitive to wheat or gluten-containing foods, consider alternative grains such as rice, millet, buckwheat (soba), and quinoa.

◆ Whenever possible, eat cooked foods and drink beverages warm or at room temperature.

◆ Drink at least eight glasses of water (64 oz.) per day. You need extra water if you consume caffeinated beverages or products or alcoholic drinks. You can make water more flavorful by adding a sprig of peppermint, or a slice of lemon, lime, or cucumber.

◆ To minimize your sugar intake, dilute fruit juices with water and avoid soft drinks.

◆ Enjoy your food. S-l-o-w down, and chew your food thoroughly.

◆ Begin meals with a prayer, an expression of thanks, or a moment of silence.

Get Enough Protein

It's essential that people with immune and autoimmune conditions get enough protein. Protein is part of every cell in the body, and is used to maintain immune function, as well as the cells of the muscles, tendons, and ligaments. All body tissues, functions, and processes involve proteins.

For clients experiencing fatigue we often recommend protein in the form of meat, poultry, or fish three or more times per day. For clients who are not able to, or do not like to eat that much animal source protein we suggest protein shakes. The most popular shakes on the market are milk-based products such as casein and whey. These products can be manufactured so that protein is maximized and fat is minimized; however, many people are dairy intolerant and therefore cannot use these products.

Soy has many health benefits including reduced heart disease and menopausal symptoms, but like milk products, soy products can cause digestive disturbances. Protein shakes can also be made out of rice protein and pea protein. While less available, these products can be easier to digest than milk- and soy-based products, so I like them the best.

The best protein sources are animal products such as meat and fish. Try eating small amounts of meat or fish with every meal. In many Asian countries, meat is often stir-fried with vegetables. In this way, the flavoring and protein of meat are combined with the health benefits of vegetables.

People with increased needs for protein—such as those who are athletic, are large size, have frequent infections, or have cancer—may do well to eat up to six protein-rich meals or snacks a day. Omega-3-rich fish, such as wild salmon, are an ideal source of protein for most people. If you have a kidney condition, you have different nutritional needs, and therefore need to seek professional advice.

Moderate amounts of lean meat that is boiled or baked are easily digestible. Some patients tolerate organic meat from naturally grazed animals, rather than commercially raised animals that are often given antibiotics and hormones. People with chronic immune disorders should not eat meat rare and should always be certain that their meat is thoroughly cooked to avoid ingesting harmful bacteria. Pork and beef are the biggest risks for bacteria. According to Dr. J. C. Breneman, author of *Basics of Food Allergy,* symptoms of bacterial infection may take up to forty-eight hours to develop. Eating shellfish is much more likely to result in bacterial infection than freshwater fish.[19]

To Be or Not to Be a Vegetarian

Many people think they're doing their body good by being a vegetarian, but that's not always the case. The fast pace of modern life is demanding, and it takes adequate protein to keep up. If you have a religious or heritage reason for being vegetarian, and your health is fine, it makes sense to keep your vegetarian diet. But many Americans who grew up on meat and potatoes—large portions, largely fried—adopt vegetarianism as a rejection of what they grew up with.

If you're a vegetarian with a troubling health condition, you may want to reevaluate your diet. To get energy, many vegetarians eat too many refined carbohydrates—starchy and sugary foods—when they would be better off with a little animal protein. Too many refined carbohydrates can lead to other problems. In our clinic, we recommend that people consider incorporating meat into their diet in reasonable 3 oz., deck-of-cards-sized servings, incorporated into soups, stews, and stir-fries, and to think of meat more as a seasoning, rather than the centerpiece of a meal.

Additionally, soy products are a staple of vegetarian diets, but in my experience 10–25 percent of Caucasians are soy intolerant. According to Chinese medicine, tofu is cool in nature, and in traditional Asian cuisine it is always cooked and mixed with ginger and other warming spices. In vegetarian restaurants here in the U.S., you're likely to eat soy in forms that are too cooling, such as raw tofu.

Eat Like a Hunter-Gatherer

"Including lean meats, more fruits and vegetables at the expense of cereal grains is a good starting point for improving nutrition," says Loren Cordain, a Colorado State University exercise physiology professor and expert on Paleolithic nutrition. According to Cordain, fossil records indicate that humans ate a very different diet ten thousand years ago than we eat today. Settling down on farms actually led to a reduction in human life span. When people started farming, and eating grains and legumes, they experienced an increase in all sorts of ills, including infant mortality, infectious diseases, iron deficiency anemia, bone mineral disorders, dental cavities, and enamel defects.

Hunters and gatherers didn't eat grains or much in the way of carbohydrates at all. In fact, they mostly ate meat. According to Cordain, the Paleolithic diet virtually turns the FDA's nutritional pyramid on its head. A survey of ethnographic data from 181 hunter-gatherer societies worldwide indicates that the average hunter-gatherer diet is 35 percent plant and 65 percent animal, "in contrast to the low-fat, high-carbohydrate, plant-based diet which is almost universally recommended by modern day nutritionists."[20]

Heal Your Leaky Gut

Our gastrointestinal lining serves to protect us against harmful bacteria, viruses, fungi, and parasites, and helps the body absorb essential nutrients. It may be damaged by drugs, particularly antibiotics, as well as by the consumption of alcohol, sugar, and fats. Holistic health professionals believe that once the gastrointestinal lining is damaged, partially digested food molecules and other toxins can enter the bloodstream, causing an autoimmune reaction. This reaction may lead to digestive disorders, rheumatoid arthritis, psoriasis, lupus, eczema, and migraine headaches.

Many people with untreatable digestive symptoms have obtained relief by following a diet that restricts yeast, sugar, and alcohol, and by taking anti-fungal herbs and medications. If your digestive disorder began after drinking from a stream, or visiting a developing country, consult with your health professional about testing and treatment for parasites.

Under the guidance of an herbalist or other holistic health professional, herbal formulas can be administered to rid the body of unhealthy pathogens. Probiotic supplements, such as acidophilus and bifidus, can be used to introduce healthy bacteria into your gut, and fructooligosaccharides (FOS) and colostrum to help normalize your gastrointestinal system. Specific dietary supplements can correct nutrient deficiencies, and herbal and vegetable enzymes can be used to help food assimilate more easily (see "Parasites" section in Chapter Three).

Identify Food Triggers / Be Aware of Food Cravings / Identify Sensitivities with a Food Diary

There is no such thing as a "best" diet. The best diet is the one that works best for you. If you have an immune disorder, you may be more sensitive to certain foods than most people. Although there are some foods that commonly cause problems, it's most important that you pay attention to your body and become familiar with its likes and dislikes. Paying attention to your body is the key to finding the best diet for you.

Food sensitivities can cause a variety of symptoms, including joint pain, digestive upset, and skin rashes and inflammation. The foods in the Sensitivity/Substitutes table below are widely known to trigger a variety of symptoms. You may find after eliminating one or more of these foods that your symptoms are reduced. It's important to go at least one week, and preferably two weeks, without a food to determine whether or not it is the cause of the symptoms. Preservatives, flavorings, processing aids, nutritional additives, and even cookware may also trigger digestive symptoms. Therefore, your diet should emphasize fresh foods whenever possible. (A complete digestive clearing plan is found in Chapter Four.)

People often force themselves to eat foods they assume are good for them, not making the connection between unpleasant symptoms and the "healthy" foods they're eating. For example, nearly all Americans assume that salads are good for them. In terms of Chinese medicine, however, salads are cold in property and should not be eaten by people with weak digestive systems. This is particularly true during the winter months, when the weather may have adverse consequences on one's health. Salads are also contraindicated in terms of Western medicine during gastrointestinal flare-ups, because they contain roughage. In practical terms, this means that some individuals can never eat salads and must have all vegetables cooked, while some can eat salads in the summer but not in winter, and others can eat salads only with the help of the herbal and dietary supplements mentioned in this book. Still others find that warming spices such as black pepper and fennel are helpful in offsetting the cold property of salads.

Food cravings are desires for food that may not be the best for us. Common cravings include chocolate and other sweets, fried foods, dairy products, spices, and acidic foods such as tomato sauce. If you notice that any of these foods give you symptoms, ask yourself, What does this food provide? For example, many of us equate sweets with nurturing because our mothers often gave us sweets as a reward, for special occasions, or to help us ease disappointments. Is there something you could be doing that would be more satisfying than eating these foods? Perhaps you could take a nap, go to a concert or movie, or simply do nothing.

If you suspect that you might have some food sensitivities, keeping a food diary can help you identify the foods your body doesn't tolerate well, as well as the ones that make you feel really good.

- ◆ Record the date, time, what you ate, and any discomfort you experience during the day.
- ◆ Rate that discomfort on a scale of 0 to 10, 0 being no discomfort, 10 being unbearable discomfort.
- ◆ See if you can attach an emotion to the discomfort, and make note of it, even if you're not sure what emotion you're feeling. Are you angry, sad, overwhelmed, anxious, fearful, grief stricken?

Wheat/Gluten Intolerance

Wheat and other gluten-containing foods can be harmful to immune function. Foods containing gluten include wheat, oats,

Sensitivity	Substitute
Milk and other dairy products	Lactaid milk, goat milk, rice milk, nut milk
Coffee and other caffeinated drinks	Green tea, herbal tea, coffee substitute
Sugar, fructose, fruit juice	Honey, whole fruit, real maple syrup, rice syrup
Eggs (chicken)	Eggs from turkey, duck, ostrich, turtle; egg substitute (made from potato)
Corn	Blue corn, alternate grains
Wheat	Rice, buckwheat, corn, quinoa
Soy	Miso or tempeh may be tolerable
Tomato, pepper, eggplant, potato	Other vegetables
Chocolate	Carob
Alcoholic beverages	Alcohol-free wine and beer, herbal relaxants
Fermented foods	Herbs and spices as seasonings
Meat and freshwater fish	Organic meat that does not contain antibiotics or hormones
Aluminum cookware	Ceramic, glass

Scale of 1 to 10, 10 being the most discomfort, and 0 being the least barley, rye, malt, triticale, spelt, and kamut. Many people with immune disorders find they have fewer digestive symptoms, more energy, and less pain if they avoid wheat and other gluten-containing food. For example, one of our clients experienced symptoms that resembled multiple sclerosis and rheumatoid arthritis, although biomedical tests were inconclusive. After two weeks on a gluten-free diet, all her joint pain disappeared, and she had more energy. Wheat sensitivity, also known as gluten intolerance, is known to cause or contribute to digestive disorders, autoimmune disease, asthma, psoriasis, diabetes, arthritis, fatigue, migraine, dermatitis herpetiformis, depression, anemia, kidney disease, osteoporosis, liver disease, and female infertility.

In gluten intolerance, the immune system reacts to gluten, a component of wheat and other grains, in the small intestine, damaging the villi and thus hampering nutrient absorption. Advanced gluten intolerance is known as celiac disease. A blood test is used to identify people who are most likely to have celiac disease, possibly followed by a biopsy of a tiny bit of intestinal tissue to check for damage to the villi. However, according to gastroenterologist Kenneth Fine, M.D., "Even though recent research has shown that celiac disease is much more common than previously suspected, affecting 1 in 100–200 Americans and Europeans, past and emerging evidence indicates that it accounts for only a small portion of the broader gluten-sensitive clinical perspective, often referred to as the 'tip of the gluten sensitive iceberg.'" At Dr. Fine's lab EnteroLab (EnteroLab.com), advanced testing that includes genetics and fat microscopy is available, in order to find out if you are intolerant to gluten. If you have blood relatives with a history of diabetes, autoimmune disease, alcoholism, and of Northern European ancestry, it is more likely that you could have gluten intolerance.

Whereas some experts believe in total avoidance, others suggest a period of gluten avoidance, followed by minimal use (once per week) of gluten-containing products. The digestive clearing plan (see Chapter Four) includes an elimination diet that avoids gluten-containing foods. You can follow this yourself whether or not you pursue medical tests.

Milk and Dairy Products

Milk can lead to a broad spectrum of complaints and is probably the most common cause of food intolerance. Milk can give rise to intestinal gas, diarrhea, heartburn, dyspepsia, stomatitis, gallbladder attacks, pancreatitis, Crohn's and colitis flare-ups, duodenal ulcer, and hemorrhoids. Other manifestations of milk intolerance are asthma, bedwetting, migraine, and hay fever. The constant use of milk and other dairy products, especially in childhood, gradually weakens the digestive system and leads to the above-mentioned symptoms.

Milk is a problem because it contains lactose. Under normal circumstances, lactose is broken down into glucose and galactose by the enzyme lactase. If the body is unable to digest and absorb lactose, it remains in the intestines, where it interferes with normal intestinal bacteria, thus leading to cramps, gas, bloating, and diarrhea. Lactose intolerance is more common among older people and in non–Northern Europeans. You can experiment with lactase drops or supplements. Some milk already has lactase in it. I am one of the many people who is not lactose intolerant according to medical tests, but who cannot tolerate milk. In fact, humans are the only animals who as adults drink milk! Some people are able to tolerate goat milk, but not cow milk. Dairy products include milk, butter, cream, butterfat, powered or condensed milk, whey, yogurt, cheese, ice cream, casein (a component of milk also referred to as caseinate), lactose, lactate, nonfat milk solids, and lactalbumin (another component of milk).

Sweets, Sugars, and Artificial Sweeteners

Most people think in terms of sweets as candy, but soft drinks are the largest source of sweetness in the standard American diet. Added sweeteners can also come in baked goods, fruit drinks, desserts, cereals, lunch meats, sauces, salad dressing, baby foods, snacks, protein bars, and even diet supplements. Restaurant food and packaged food contain more sugars than home cooking, because sugar sells.

Traditionally, our ancestors' access to sweet foods was limited to honey and fruit. Sugarcane is a tropical grass that was first cultivated in New Guinea. In the 1700s, millions of slaves were used to work in the sugarcane fields to feed Europe's sugar habit.

According to the USDA, Americans consumed 147 pounds of sweeteners per person in 2001. These sweeteners include sugar, sucrose, fructose, saccharin (Sweet 'N Low), Aspartame (Nutra-Sweet, Equal), sucralose (Splenda), and acesulfame-K (Sunett). Consumption of high fructose corn syrup (HFCS) has exploded since its introduction in the late '60s, and this highly absorbable sweetener is known to cause insulin resistance and diabetes. Our increased consumption of sugar contributes to the common ailments of our day, including obesity, inflammation, diabetes, hypertension, high cholesterol levels, and immune dysfunction. In Chinese medicine, excessive consumption of sweeteners—both natural and artificial sweeteners—is seen as causing damp and heat symptoms.

Eating sweeteners also reduces your appetite for nutrient-dense foods such as protein, fruits, and vegetables. To promote optimal immune health, eat mostly fresh fruits, vegetables, and lean sources of protein. Substitute water—by itself or with a slice of lemon, lime, or cucumber—for soft drinks. If you must have a sweet, try to enjoy it as a treat, not a daily routine.

82

All sweets including artificial sweeteners can cause digestive symptoms. Chocolate can give rise to immediate reactions such as diarrhea, and can cause migraine, acne, enuresis, nasal congestion, pruritus, urticaria (hives), stomatitis, and allergic rhinitis. Diet sodas are dangerous chemical cocktails that, in my opinion, should be avoided by everyone.

Fruit and Fruit Juices

Orange and other citrus foods should be tested separately. Oranges are a common allergen, but people who are allergic to oranges may or may not be allergic to other citrus fruits. Common symptoms are nasal congestion, heartburn, dyspepsia, and canker sores. Fruit juices are too concentrated—after all, you wouldn't eat eight oranges in one sitting, the equivalent of which is contained in many juices! Fruit juices also increase the sugar and acid load of the digestive tract.

Alcohol

Some individuals have varying sensitivities to beer, red or white wine, and other forms of alcohol. Some patients are able to tolerate preservative-free beer and wine, others hard alcohol, since they don't contain preservatives. Alcohol is contraindicated for those who have a hot condition (see Introduction).

Coffee and Caffeinated Beverages

Caffeinated beverages damage the digestive tract. Coffee is very acidic and can cause many digestive symptoms. Coffee reacts with chocolate and cola and can lead to gastritis, migraine headaches, and joint pain.

How to Get Off Caffeine

Stopping coffee or other caffeinated beverages "cold turkey" can cause you to experience lethargy, depression, severe headaches, nausea, and even muscle and joint pain. This is why I suggest withdrawing slowly, cutting out caffeinated sodas first, and substituting tea, which is easier to digest, for coffee. Instead of drinking full cups of coffee or tea, mix your coffee or tea with decaf, increasing this amount until you are using all decaf. You may even try putting a grain of coffee or a couple of drops of tea under your tongue. Try *Vrooom* (Adrenosen), a formula I developed that can be used concurrently to help give a "pick-me-up." Homeopathic remedies may also be useful for caffeine withdrawal.

Aluminum Cookware

Such cookware can cause digestive upset, gas, and constipation. It has also been implicated in Alzheimer's disease. If you use aluminum cookware, throw it out! Aluminum canned foods can be equally as bad. Ceramic, glass, and enamel cookware are best; stainless steel is also acceptable.

Soy

Many people have intolerance to soybeans and other soy products such as tofu and soy sauce. Restaurants, especially fast-food chains, cook with soy oil and flour. Soy flour is also used by bakers in breads, cakes, rolls, and pastries. Some crackers contain soybean flour. Salad dressings often contain soybean oil.

Asian Restaurant Syndrome

The problem with the Asian diet for non-Asians is that it contains soy products such as teriyaki and soy sauce, which many Americans are allergic to. The Asian diet also consists of many fermented foods, which are contraindicated for those who have candida complex (candidiasis). A further problem is MSG (monosodium glutamate), which can lead to upset stomach, thirst, dizziness, headaches, tiredness, high blood pressure, and rashes.

Corn

Corn is difficult to avoid as it is ubiquitous in manufactured foods. Some patients are able to tolerate fresh corn off the cob, but not canned corn or other forms of corn and cornmeal. While corn can cause acute reactions, it is more likely to gradually weaken the digestive system, leading to symptoms such as gastritis, colitis, allergic rhinitis (hay fever), asthma, migraine, and hives. Corn is found in Mexican food and chips, and in alcoholic beverages including beer, ale, brandy, gin, whiskey, and vodka. It may be contained in wines, including the sparkling variety. Dextrose is corn sugar and glucose is corn syrup. Corn is found in talcum powder, bath oils and powders, and clothing starch.

Nuts and Peanuts

Nuts are high in fat and cause allergic reactions in millions of Americans. Peanuts and peanut butter are a frequent cause of dyspepsia and migraine; technically peanuts are legumes not nuts.

Yeast and Fermented Foods

Yeast is commonly used in food preparation. It converts sugars to alcohol and carbon dioxide in a fermentation process. Yeast and mold may lead to cross-reactivity in some hypersensitive people. Sauerkraut, vinegar, and miso may aggravate digestive symptoms.

Eggs

Eggs can give rise to gallbladder flare-ups, gastritis, dyspepsia, migraine, asthma, diarrhea, acne, and hives. Eggs are often contaminated with salmonella, which can cause a host of digestive disorders and even sore joints. Powdered eggs are of particular risk for salmonella. Therefore, egg dishes must be heated thoroughly to 160°F (71.2°C). In addition, *do not eat raw eggs!* Eggs may also contain pesticide residues, antibiotics, and hormones. Some individuals are allergic only to the egg white, not the yolk. Albumin, livetin, ovomucin, ovomucoid, and vitellin indicate the presence of eggs or egg components. People who are sensitive to chicken eggs might try substituting duck, goose, turkey, ostrich, or turtle eggs.

Change Your Oil

Numerous studies have shown that people who eat fish such as salmon and sardines, or take fish oil supplements, have a lower incidence of heart disease, dementia, certain kinds of cancer, asthma, diabetes, psoriasis, and allergies. Fish oil has been studied for its effect on conditions such as depression, PMS, rheumatoid arthritis, colitis, and attention-deficit/hyperactivity disorder

Examples of Fish with High Levels of Fats and Omega-3 Fatty Acids.

Amounts shown are percentage of the uncooked fish, as presented typically in shops.

FISH	% TOTAL FAT	% OMEGA-3 FATTY ACIDS
Mackerel (Atlantic)	13.9	2.3
Albacore tuna	7.2	2.1
Herring (Atlantic)	18.0	1.6
Salmon (Atlantic)	6.3	1.4
Lake trout	9.4	1.4
Chinook salmon	10.4	1.4
Bluefin tuna	4.9	1.2
Striped bass	2.3	0.8
Bluefish	4.2	0.8
Smelt	2.4	0.7
Rainbow trout	3.4	0.6
Swordfish	4.0	0.6
Pollack	1.0	0.4
Halibut	2.3	0.4
Freshwater catfish	4.3	0.4

Sources: itmonline.org; fareshare.net/fish

Tips for Using Fish Oil

- Be sure the fish oil is not rancid. The best supplements include a small amount of vitamin E to prevent rancidity.
- Take fish oil capsules with food, or consider taking fish oil capsules with digestive enzymes, to prevent burping or gastrointestinal burning.
- Experiment with different brands. In our clinic, we recommend Neptune krill oil, or cod-liver oil, or fish oil capsules that are enterically coated to make it digestion easier.
- Make sure your fish oil has been tested for mercury and other heavy metals.
- Be aware that high-dosage fish oil may increase bleeding time and should be used only under professional supervision if you are taking anticoagulant medications like Coumadin (warfarin).

(ADHD). Fish oil reduces platelet aggregation, helping to prevent clots from sticking to the walls of blood vessels, and also decreases triglyceride synthesis and suppresses inflammation.

Fish oils are so good for us because they contain essential omega-3 fatty acids EPA (eicosapentaenoic acid) and DHA (docosahexaenoic acid), which are known to protect against a long list of chronic diseases. EPA and DHA appear to reduce leukotrienes, interleukin-2, and tumor necrosis factor. In addition, DHA is essential to healthy brain and retina function. EPA and DHA are found in plankton, a diet staple for many sea animals. EPA and DHA are found in high amounts in wild salmon, herring, cod, mackerel, and sardines. EPA and DHA can also be found in supplements and cod-liver oil. Neptune krill oil offers many advantages over other fish oil sources of EPA and DHA, because krill oil is free of toxic heavy metals, offers a more concentrated dose of EPA and DHA, thus requiring fewer pills per day, is a stronger antioxidant, and is much less likely to cause digestive upset.

Other healthful oils include olive oil for cooking, and sesame, avocado, walnut, and flax oil in dressings. By increasing your intake of ocean fish, taking fish oil supplements, and incorporating other healthy oils into your diet, you can lessen inflammation and protect your brain and heart.

The Energetic Effects of Foods and Herbs

In Chinese medicine, foods and herbs are classified according to their energetic effects. Every substance, whether a Twinkie or chicken or a medicinal herb, has a particular effect on the body. For example, like a lot of junk food, Twinkies are sweet, and thus dampening and heating. In Chinese medicine, too much sweet creates damp, which can then transform into heat.

Modern processing practices complicate the picture a bit. The energetic quality of animal products depends a lot on how they're processed. Free-range chickens are less warming than chickens that have been shot up with a lot of antibiotics, like most grocery store chickens. How was that animal raised? Did it live in a coop with other diseased birds, or was it allowed to roam freely?

Vegetables, too, have a history that influences their effect on the body. In an ideal world, we'd all grow our own vegetables, using no pesticides or other chemicals, but instead nourishing our gardens with our own Qi and intention. There's a joy in eating carrots that we've watered, and weeded, and talked to, that's different from eating carrots bought at the grocery store. For those of us who aren't quite ready to tend our own vegetable garden, however, a middle step toward more nourishing produce is to buy organic directly from small growers at a farmers' market.

Drink Plenty of Water

Dehydration is common in Western industrialized countries. Many people drink caffeinated beverages such as coffee, tea, or soda, which have a diuretic action that can lead to dehydration. Alcohol and chemicals in diet soda also increase the body's need for water. I recommend that you drink five glasses per day of water, preferably at room temperature, or hot (with lemon or lime); and three cups a day of peppermint tea, or chamomile or ginger tea for a cold condition (see description or "Cold" condition in table in Introduction). Hot water or herbal tea is particularly beneficial before meals. Average sized persons need eight to ten glasses per day, while overweight and large-build people need ten to twelve glasses daily.

Fats

Fats can cause diarrhea, gas, bloating, and belching more than other foods, so following a low-fat diet is important if you have a chronic digestive disorder. However, not all fats are to be avoided. Try to use oils like olive or canola (unsaturated fat) that are liquid, rather than butter (saturated fat), which is solid at room temperature. Studies conducted in Denmark and Japan indicate that persons whose diets contain both omega-3 and omega-6 oils have a much lower incidence of inflammatory disease. Omega-6 oils are found in corn, sunflower, and soy oils, as well as in animal fat. In order to increase our ratio of omega-3 oils, we can eat more fish, avocados, flax, canola, rapeseed, and sesame seed oils, or take supplemental EPA. The following fish contain healthy omega-3 oils: salmon, mackerel, anchovy, cod, striped bass, snapper, haddock, sardine, trout, tuna, and sablefish.

Pearl Barley (Coix)

Pearl barley is used in traditional Chinese medicine to treat the digestive system. It is highly recommended for people who have digestive disorders, and is a part of the digestive clearing diet. Porridge can be made by using 1 cup of pearl barley to 4 to 6 cups of water. Pearl barley gets rid of dampness and is thought to benefit the immune system.

Rice

The eighty-four-year-old herbalist with whom I practice recommends a bowl of rice with each meal for people with chronic digestive disorders, as rice is one of the most digestible foods. Also consider having a soup consisting of chicken, vegetable, and rice, or rice porridge, made with 1 cup of rice cooked in 4 to 6 cups of water. White rice is easier to digest, while brown rice is more nutritious. In addition, winter squash, carrot, rutabaga, parsnip, turnip, sweet potato, pumpkin, onion, leek, celery, scallion, white pepper, umeboshi plum, and cooked greens are all considered good foods for the digestive system.

Avoid Restaurants and Fast Food

What's so bad about restaurants? The problem with restaurants, even restaurants that serve healthy foods, is you do not know what is really in each recipe, so it's impossible to anticipate what your reaction may be to eating a restaurant meal. Furthermore, restaurant food is almost always higher in fat and sweeteners than food you would cook at home, since the emphasis is more on taste than on nutrition. Often, we make less wise choices when eating out. Another problem with restaurants is that food may not be properly cooked or stored, and spoiled food may even be used. Finally, restaurant employees do not always follow regulations about hygiene, and may spread parasites, viruses, or bacteria.

Eliminate Smoking, Alcohol, and Sweets

The alcoholic, the cigarette or marijuana smoker, and the modern office worker who eats chocolate or other sweets have more in common than you may think. All of these habits contribute to low blood sugar, medically known as hypoglycemia. Hypoglycemia can cause many digestive symptoms such as constant hunger, craving for sweets, gastrointestinal pain, food cravings, and indigestion, in addition to fatigue, depression, irritability, and headaches. According to some nutritionists, it is possible to have symptoms of low blood sugar even though all medical tests are normal. In his book *Low Blood Sugar,* Dr. Martin Budd writes, "I find that many patients suffering from stomach ulcers, heartburn, hiatal hernia, and other digestive ailments often have a blood sugar imbalance." Low blood sugar can be corrected by the following measures:[21]

- Avoid sugar, sweets, and artificial sweeteners.
- Eliminate alcohol, smoking, and recreational drugs.
- Eat protein in the morning.
- Use protein or whole fruits to counter sweet cravings.
- Eat four to six light meals per day.

Create a Health Care Team

Chronic disease can make you feel powerless; taking control of your health can help you feel empowered. Select health professionals who have empathy as well as skill. It may not be realistic to expect to find a compassionate doctor who is also the most up-to-date on the latest research. Choose the balance that feels the most comfortable to you.

Most medical doctors are not aware of the breadth of natural medicine. One of my clients, after experiencing great results at our clinic, wondered why his medical doctor had never told him about the benefits of herbs. I explained that if you want a diagnosis and treatment based on Western medicine, you go to a Western medical doctor. If you want herbs for your condition, you have to go to an herbalist.

Whether you see a medical doctor or a holistic practitioner, here are some suggestions to make the most of your visits:

- Make a list of questions before meeting with your health professional. Let him or her know at the beginning of the meeting that you have questions. Inquire about costs, treatment and diagnostic options, and risks and side effects associated with drugs and surgery. What length of time should I expect before I see results? What are the possible consequences of delaying medication or surgery in order to try natural healing methods? Can surgery or toxic drugs

Meditation with Breath

Sit or lie down with your spine straight.
Follow the directions below. Twenty
minutes once or twice per day should be
enough to reduce tension and improve
your alertness and energy level. Over time
your skin will thank you.

- Place one hand on your abdomen
  covering your navel.
- Inhale through your nose, being
  conscious of your abdomen
  extending; it may be helpful to
  repeatedly say to yourself "breathe
  deeply" during inhalation.
- Hold your breath for a comfortable
  period, then exhale slowly through
  your mouth, paying attention to your
  abdomen deflating; again, it may be
  helpful to say "relax completely"
  during exhalation.
- An alternative is the "four times four
  breath." Breathe in for a count of four. Hold your breath for a count of
  four, then let your breath out for a count of four. Continue breathing
  in this fashion for twenty minutes. A more advanced version is to
  breathe in for a count of four, hold for four, breathe out for four, and
  hold your breath with your lungs empty for a count of four before
  breathing in.

(such as chemotherapy) be scheduled after, rather than
before, my vacation? Are there new or experimental treatments that might help me? Could the procedure you
suggest be done with a less invasive method? Is this the best
place to get treated? Searching for the most experienced
professional is a good idea if your case is difficult.

- Don't hide your symptoms. Although you may be embarrassed to talk about some of your symptoms, it's important
  to be as specific as possible. All too often patients wait until

the end of the visit to convey the most important
information.

◆ If you are meeting with a holistic health professional,
explain when your symptoms began, and tell them what
you think the cause is. If you have any unhealthy habits
that could be contributing to your health problem, it is
crucial that you bring these up, as your practitioner may
have helpful suggestions.

Instant Stress Reduction

1. Exercise.
2. Do the 4 x 4 breathing, or the abdominal self-massage
   mentioned earlier in this chapter.
3. Get perspective: pretend you are looking at yourself and all your
   troubles from an airplane twenty thousand feet in the air.
4. Perspective #2: Play a forward and backward movie of the
   stressful event in your mind. Experiment with various fast
   forward and reverse speeds.
5. Apply lavender or other soothing essential oils to your inside
   wrists and inhale deeply. Take relaxing herbs such as kava,
   valerian, or passionflower or lemon balm tea.
6. Spell out the letters and repeat the following phrase very *slowly:*
   "S-L-O-W D-O-W-N, R-E-L-A-X."
7. Think about all the things you are grateful for.
8. Draw a stick figure with a balloon above it; write your stressful
   thoughts inside the cartoon balloon.
9. Make a half smile by curling up the corners of your lips.
10. Rub your heart clockwise and repeat something encouraging or
    inspiring to yourself.
11. Take a bath or hot shower.
12. Act like the person you want to be.

- If possible, bring your spouse or a friend with you. Companions can help reduce your anxiety in the waiting room, can help you remember to ask certain questions during your appointment, and can accompany you to a meal or favorite activity afterward.

Remember that health professionals are human. If they do something you don't like, share your feelings. It is always more productive to make "I feel" statements rather than statements such as, "You did this.... You don't care about me." If you are unable to speak up, consider writing a letter to your health professional.

In addition to your medical doctor, you may want to see a specialist in one of the following areas. Ask a friend or colleague for a referral or you may write to me (see Resource Guide) for a health professional who practices herbology.

- **Herbalist:** Look for an herbalist who practices full time or who has another specialty, such as acupuncture. Feel free to ask about his or her training; the usual training consists of either formal academic training or apprenticeship. It has been my experience that properly recommended herbs can make a great difference in immune health. An herbalist should offer dietary and lifestyle counseling, and may or may not be knowledgeable about dietary supplements.
- **Nutritional Counselor:** Herbalists, nutritionists, acupuncturists, and medical doctors practice nutritional counseling. A nutritionist can offer suggestions about diet as well as lifestyle changes, and recommend specific dietary supplements. Dietitians are knowledgeable about meal plans, but they are usually not healers.
- **Acupuncturist:** Acupuncture involves inserting hair-thin needles into the body at specific points, and benefits overall energy flow as mapped out by the ancient Chinese.

Acupuncture can be quite helpful in relieving pain, but its ability to treat other conditions should not be overlooked. I recommend seeing an acupuncturist who also practices herbology.

◆ **Chiropractor:** Chiropractic was developed in 1895 by Daniel David Palmer, a self-taught healer in Iowa, who believed that many ailments were caused by vertebrae pressing on spinal nerves and interfering with nerve transmission, which he called "subluxations." Most chiropractic practitioners today combine spinal adjustments with nutritional counseling and exercise recommendations. Try to find a chiropractor who uses gentle techniques—high-velocity maneuvers can be contraindicated especially for seniors and people who are not constitutionally robust. If you're weak or elderly, or find your condition doesn't improve with chiropractic, consider acupuncture or osteopathy, which tend to be gentler than spinal adjustments.

◆ **Hypnotherapist:** A hypnotherapist can help you break the bad habits that may be contributing to your disorder, and can give you suggestions for coping with your symptoms.

◆ **Massage Therapist:** Therapeutic massage can be very relaxing. A skilled therapist can move energy through the body's channels in a manner similar to acupuncture.

◆ **Therapist:** Because the mind and body are linked, a therapist can teach you how to cope with your disorder. Look for a therapist who is result-oriented and has experience with chronic diseases.

◆ **Osteopath:** Osteopaths (D.O.s) attend four years of medical school, just like M.D.s, and practice standard Western medicine, but they also receive additional training in hands-on manipulation and the musculoskeletal system.

Osteopathic manipulative therapy (OMT) is a gentle therapy in which the practitioner applies a very small amount of pressure to promote healthy movement and release compressed bones and joints. Look for an osteopath trained in OMT.

Take Inventory of What You're Taking

People who are dealing with an immune condition typically get prescribed many medications. We often see clients who are taking several different prescription drugs and over-the-counter (OTC) medications, along with various teas, supplements, vitamins, and other products. I believe that taking too many substances can decrease their effectiveness. Oftentimes when clients are taking multiple medications and supplements they don't take therapeutic dosages. This is similar to forgetting to take one's medication. If you forget to take your medication it will not work.

There are millions of people in the U.S. taking supplements and medications they don't need. A good herbalist can help clients sort out exactly what they're taking, and point out drugs that may no longer be necessary, or that can be decreased or eliminated through herbs, diet, and lifestyle. For example, Mark initially came in taking two different blood-pressure medications and a cholesterol-lowering medication. In addition, a holistic doctor had recommended he take garlic and Co Q-10. Over the next nine months, I worked with Mark with herbs and lifestyle and dietary counseling. In that time, Mark lost twenty pounds, and no longer required any medication. Had he not been monitored at our clinic, Mark might not have thought to see his doctor about eliminating the medications. It's a good idea to take inventory with your health professional every six months, to make sure there's a good reason to keep taking what you're taking.

When you see your health professional, be sure to discuss whether you tend to be sensitive, or hypersensitive, to medications and herbs. You may be considered hypersensitive if you have allergies or reactions, and tend to respond to low dosages of medications and herbs. On the other hand, you may be hyposensitive if you generally need higher doses of medications, or need to try several different approaches before you find one that works. Individuals on several medications often do not respond as well to alternative approaches as individuals who are not heavily medicated.

Make a list of any medications you are taking. Look them up in the *Physician's Desk Reference (PDR)* or *Nurse's Drug Guide,* available at a public library or bookstore. Find out if any of these medications have side effects. Meet with your physician, pharmacist, and holistic health professional to find out if there are alternatives to these medications that won't cause unpleasant side effects. Before starting on any drugs, you should know about their risks.

Question Medical Tests and Procedures

Make an informed decision by doing your own research and reading up on any medical tests or procedures your doctor may recommend. Information is available through libraries as well as the internet. Whenever possible, get a second opinion before undergoing any surgery or procedure for a chronic illness. In some cases, such as barium enemas, the risks may outweigh the benefits. Many surgeries aren't medically necessary, and surgery doesn't guarantee that you will be without symptoms. Countless persons undergo operations that only temporarily relieve their problems. Also, inappropriate surgery can spread cancer growth.

Testing makes sense if something is wrong, but if you are having no symptoms, the risks and benefits of all tests should be carefully weighed. While the Western medical establishment assumes that screening healthy people for cancer and other diseases saves lives, "The evidence shows that some screening tests are much more useful than others," according to Dr. Barnett Kramer of the National Institutes of Health (NIH).[22] Doctors have financial and legal incentives for recommending tests. Some testing is helpful. For example, Pap smears for cervical cancer and screenings for colon cancer are worthwhile procedures that have decreased mortality for these cancers. The value of other tests may be questionable.

One of the problems with screening healthy people is that medical tests may reveal malignant tumors, but they may also show growths that are not harmful, and subject patients to needless operations and medical procedures, not to mention emotional turmoil. According to Dr. Steven H. Woolf, a professor and member of the U.S. Preventive Services Task Force, "Patients have little idea of the risk that awaits them regarding screening tests."[23]

Some of the more questionable tests include mammography for breast cancer, blood tests for early signs of prostate cancers, and spiral CT scans for spotting lung cancer. Prostate-specific antigen (PSA) testing can lead to the detection of minute tumors, but most prostate cancers grow so slowly that patients typically die of something else, and aggressive prostate cancer can't be stopped with existing orthodox treatments such as radiation or surgery, which may cause impotence.

Also, just because there is physical evidence of illness—on an X-ray or biopsy result—it doesn't necessarily mean there's a problem. Many people who, according to their X-ray or MRI results, should be in great pain actually feel just fine. Many people whose test results show colon polyps, hiatal hernias, or diminished brain capacity are actually functioning quite well. The opposite is also true. I often see clients whose medical tests are normal, and there is no suitable medical explanation for the way they get sick all the time, or for their pain, or for their repeated fainting spells.

Drug/Herb Interactions

When drugs and herbs interact, the result is generally to either increase or decrease their effects. Sedative herbs such as kava could be too sedating if combined with sleeping pills. Herbs can also change the length of time medications are retained in the body. For example, by speeding up the elimination process, bulking agents and laxatives reduce absorption of medications in the intestine.

In pharmacological terms, interactions fall into two general categories: *pharmacokinetic* and *pharmacodynamic.* Pharmacokinetic processes include changes in a substance's absorption, distribution, metabolism, or excretion, in turn changing the amount and duration of the availability of a substance at receptor sites. Pharmacodynamic interactions are due to changes at the receptor site itself, and may increase or decrease a substance's effect.

While the drug industry and medical doctors have overemphasized the dangers of herb/drug interactions, the true dangers are drug/drug interactions. The average senior citizen takes five or more different medications, and nobody, including the pharmaceutical companies who manufacture them, knows what those drugs do when combined. These combinations certainly haven't been proven safe or effective. It's estimated that about 100,000 people die each year from prescription drug side effects, and about 300 per year from over-the-counter medications.[24] According to a study published in the *Journal of the American Geriatrics Society*,[25] 9.4 percent of hospital admissions were due to a drug-induced illness. These patients were taking an average of 5.7 medications at the same time.

Minimizing Drug/Herb Interactions

◆ It's always best to see a health professional trained in herbology.
◆ Generally take herbs and drugs two or more hours apart.
◆ In order to minimize herb/drug interactions purchase all herbs and supplements from the health professional who is monitoring you.
◆ Make regular appointments to discuss your protocol.

Allergy Medications

Allergic rhinitis and asthma are treated with medications such as antihistamines, decongestants, and anti-inflammatory nasal sprays, along with allergen avoidance and allergy shots. Antihistamines work best for itching, sneezing, and nasal discharge, while decongestants work better for nasal stuffiness. Short-acting, over-the-counter antihistamines, including loratadine (Claritin), relieve mild to moderate symptoms, but can cause drowsiness. Check the label—ingredients that may cause drowsiness include brompheniramine, carbinoxamine, chlorpheniramine, clemastine, dexbrompheniramine, diphenhydramine, and triprolidine. Longer-acting antihistamines such as fexofenadine (Allegra) and cetirizine (Zyrtec) cause less drowsiness.

Nasal decongestant sprays, particularly the long-acting type, can cause rebound congestion if used for more than a week at a time. Anti-inflammatory nasal corticosteroid sprays such as fluticasone (Flonase), mometasone (Nasonex), and triamcinolone (Nasacort) don't cause rebound congestion and can be more effective in preventing and treating allergic rhinitis symptoms than antihistamines. Cromolyn sodium is available as a nasal spray

(Nasalcrom) for treating hay fever, and as eye drops for itchy, bloodshot eyes.

Allergy shots, also called allergy immunotherapy, desensitize the body to allergens by injecting them under the skin in weekly, increasing doses. Allergy shots are a long-term process—a full course of allergy shots can take several years to complete, and it can take a year for allergy symptoms to abate. For this reason, allergy shots are usually recommended for people with severe allergy symptoms, including anaphylaxis and extreme reactions to insect stings.[26]

Anti-Fungal Drugs

While topical anti-fungals are often more effective and less messy than herbal topical remedies, dermatologists also often prescribe anti-fungal drugs internally. While effective, drugs such as keto-conazole (Nizoral), fluconazole (Diflucan), itraconazole (Spora-nox), and terbinafine (Lamisil) are toxic to the liver and are expensive. If the fungal infection is not life-threatening, it may make sense to use pharmaceuticals for topical use, and diet and complementary approaches to treat fungus systemically.

Antibiotics

While no one denies that antibiotics are one of the greatest medical discoveries of all time, their overuse and misuse are currently a serious health problem. In fact, at a congressional hearing, evidence was presented that an estimated 40 to 60 percent of prescriptions for antibiotics in America are prescribed for the wrong conditions, or for diseases for which their use is not warranted.

A case in point are viral conditions. According to the Association for the Prudent Use of Antibiotics[27] antibiotics are not appropriate for upper respiratory infections in previously healthy adults, because these infections are usually caused by a virus. You should never insist that your doctor prescribe antibiotics for viral infections like the common cold—for a virus, you need an anti-viral medication, or rely on non-drug treatments. Antibiotics are also inappropriate for uncomplicated sinusitis and uncomplicated acute bronchitis in previously healthy adults. Antibiotics are not only over-administered to humans, but because they are used to enhance growth and prevent disease in chickens, turkeys, pigs, and cattle raised for human consumption, the meat-eaters among us are getting a double dose.

There are a number of problems with the overuse of antibiotics. Antibiotics have adverse effects on the immune system, and bacteria can develop a resistance to antibiotics, so that the antibiotics have little or no effect. This process is speeded up when you don't finish your antibiotic prescriptions. Antibiotics not only kill off the bad bacteria, but also the good bacteria that protect us from opportunistic infections. Good bacteria crowd out invading bacteria and fungi by attaching to the intestinal wall. If all the good bacteria are killed off, the bad bacteria can take over.

If you must use antibiotics, ask your health professional to take a culture and test it to make sure the correct antibiotic is used. When you are prescribed a course of antibiotics, follow instructions exactly. If you don't take all the antibiotics you're prescribed, the bacteria may not be completely killed off. So the antibiotics will no longer work for you, and you'll still have the bug in your system; the next time it breaks out, you'll need a stronger antibiotic. Taking probiotic products two days for every one day you're on antibiotics can improve immune function and reduce antibiotic side effects. Probiotics should always be taken on an empty stomach, at least two hours before or after taking an antibiotic. Unless you work in a medical office or hospital. Avoid anti-bacterial soaps and cleansers, because they kill only the weakest bacteria, allowing the strongest bacteria to thrive.

Antidepressants

Americans are taking more antidepressants than ever before, with prescriptions steadily increasing since Prozac, the first of the newer SSRI antidepressants, was approved by the FDA in 1987. The number of Americans treated for depression jumped from 1.7 million to 6.3 million between 1987 and 1997, while the percentage of those patients taking antidepressants doubled from 37 percent to 75 percent. The increase in antidepressant use stems from a variety of factors, including the aggressive marketing of the newer antidepressants and increased insurance coverage for pharmaceuticals. But studies show that the current batch of antidepressants are often not that effective, and that they can have disturbing side effects, as well as withdrawal symptoms.

While they can be beneficial, antidepressants are not a panacea, but come with negative effects that warrant serious consideration. Antidepressants are about 40 percent effective, while placebos are about 30 percent effective, so antidepressants are only slightly better than placebos in terms of effects. Studies indicate that the most effective treatment for depression combines antidepressants with cognitive behavioral therapy to change negative thinking and behaviors associated with depression. For people who are suicidal, antidepressants and ongoing counseling are called for, but if depression is mild or moderate, it's better to try herbs and supplements first. Antidepressants come with varying side effects, so if you're considering antidepressants, you'll want to do some research and decide which side effect profile you're willing to tolerate. People often report that antidepressants stop working after a time, and it can be difficult to get off antidepressants, physiologically and emotionally, requiring a very gradual reduction in dosage over a period of weeks to minimize withdrawal effects. Finally, I believe that antidepressants can hamper the healing process. While antidepressants alleviate the emotional highs and lows, I believe they numb the body as well, making it harder to see any benefits from herbs.

Serotonin and norepinephrine are crucial for good mood, and antidepressants may work by increasing the amount of serotonin and norepinephrine at the nerve endings in your brain. The earliest antidepressants, in use from the 1960s to the 1980s, were the tricyclic antidepressants and the monoamine oxidase (MAO) inhibitors.

Tricyclic antidepressants are named for their triple-ring chemical structure. Members of this group, such as amitriptyline (Elavil) and doxepin (Sinequan), work by blocking the reuptake of norepinephrine and serotonin at nerve endings, and tend to be sedating, with side effects similar to those of MAO inhibitors. The most common side effects of tricyclic antidepressants are dry mouth, constipation, bladder problems, sexual problems, blurred vision, dizziness, and drowsiness.

Monoamine oxidase inhibitors (MAOIs)—including isocarboxazid (Marplan), phenelzine (Nardil), and tranylcypromine (Parnate)—inhibit monoamine oxidase, an enzyme that breaks down norepinephrine and serotonin. Less monoamine oxidase means that more of the good mood substances are available for your brain. MAO inhibitors have a long list of side effects, including dry mouth, constipation, blurred vision, and impotence, along with more serious adverse effects like convulsions and liver damage. To avoid the risk of stroke, it's also necessary for the patient to avoid foods containing tyramine, such as certain cheeses, herring, beer, and wine. For these reasons, MAO inhibitors are generally used only for people who are not responsive to other antidepressants.

Selective serotonin reuptake inhibitors, or SSRIs—like fluoxetine (Prozac), paroxetine (Paxil), sertraline (Zoloft), and citalopram (Celexa)—were a revolution in the antidepressant world in the late 1980s because they were said to have fewer side effects than their predecessors. Common SSRI side effects include headache, nausea, nervousness, insomnia, tremors, diarrhea, dry mouth, weight loss, and sexual problems.

Newer antidepressants introduced in the 1990s included venlafaxine (Effexor) and nefazodone (Serzone), which affect both serotonin and norepinephrine, like the earlier tricyclic antidepressants. Two other newer antidepressants include mirtazapine (Remeron), which is sedating, and bupropion (Wellbutrin), which has a stimulating effect.

Trazodone (Desyrel) acts as an antidepressant, though its mechanism is not clear. Common side effects include upset stomach, diarrhea, stomach pain or gas, drowsiness, fatigue, anxiety, insomnia, nightmares, dry mouth, sensitivity to sunlight, and changes in appetite or weight.[28]

Chemotherapy/Cancer Drugs

Chemotherapy simply means the use of drugs to kill cancer cells or bacteria. Many drugs used to treat cancer have severe side effects, including nausea, vomiting, bone marrow suppression, hair loss, and skin and GI tract ulcers. Herbs and acupuncture can help ameliorate these side effects.

Before trying anti-nausea drugs, try eating small meals throughout the day so that your stomach is not empty. Snacks such as crackers or toast, as well as clear liquids, are helpful, as are tart foods such as lemons and pickles. Quiet Digestion is an herbal formula that has helped many people who suffer from the side effects of chemotherapy drugs.

Doxorubicin (Adriamycin, Doxil, and Rubex) is an antibiotic that interferes with DNA synthesis and thus inhibits cell reproduction. Side effects include nausea and vomiting after treatment, loss of appetite, diarrhea, difficulty swallowing, thinning or brittle hair, sunburn-like skin irritation, and swelling, pain, redness, or peeling of skin on the palms of the hands and soles of the feet.

Fluorouracil (Adrucil) is a pyrimidine antagonist used to treat solid tumors. It works by preventing the normal synthesis and replication of DNA. Its side effects include nausea, vomiting, gastrointestinal ulcers, bone marrow suppression, and hair loss.

Tamoxifen (Nolvadex) inhibits the growth of hormone-dependent breast tumors by blocking the estrogen receptor. Side effects resemble menopause symptoms; including nausea, hot flashes, rashes, and vaginal bleeding.

Mechlorethamine (Mustargen), also called nitrogen mustard, prevents cancer cells from reproducing by binding with DNA. Its side effects include nausea, vomiting, bone marrow suppression, hair loss, skin and GI tract ulcers, missing menstrual periods, and painful rashes.

Paclitaxel (Taxol), a drug originally derived from yew tree bark, stops cell division and is commonly used to treat ovarian and breast cancer, Kaposi's sarcoma, melanoma, and leukemia. Its side effects include bone marrow suppression and peripheral nerve problems.

Methotrexate (Folex, Rheumatrex) is used to treat abnormal cell growth and is prescribed for recalcitrant psoriasis, rheumatoid arthritis, and cancer. Methotrexate inhibits the chemical that makes folic acid, and that deficiency of folic acid in turn inhibits the synthesis of DNA, and thus the reproduction of cancer cells. Methotrexate is toxic to the liver and can cause suppression of the bone marrow, rashes, fatigue, fever, gastrointestinal problems, and lung complications. Methotrexate works by depleting folic acid, so if you are taking this medication, ask your health professional about supplementing with folic acid (400 to 800 mcg. per day). Because it is so toxic, tests should be administered to measure liver and kidney function while you are on methotrexate.

Immunosuppressive Drugs

Autoimmune disorders are most commonly treated with steroids, though severe allergic reactions and immune diseases—such as multiple sclerosis, myasthenia gravis, and systemic lupus erythematosus—may be treated with stronger immunosuppressant drugs such as methotrexate, cyclophosphamide, and azathioprine.

Cyclosporine and infliximab are two commonly used immunosuppressive drugs. Cyclosporine is used as a medication of last resort for severe psoriasis and other autoimmune conditions because of its severe side effects, which include blood abnormalities, tremor, convulsions, headache, insomnia, night sweats, skin malignancies, and hallucinations. About 25 percent of individuals who take cyclosporine will have some kidney damage. Less common side effects include central nervous system disturbances such as seizures. Cyclosporine inhibits the production of interleukin-2 and suppresses the helper T cells that regulate the activation of other immune cells.

Infliximab (Remicade) is approved for Crohn's disease and rheumatoid arthritis, and is undergoing studies for its use with severe psoriasis. Because it suppresses the immune system, it can predispose a patient to infections including tuberculosis and to cancer. It's also very expensive.

Interferon/Immunoglobulin Injections

Interferon is produced by the body to increase immune function. It is an anti-viral that also stimulates the immune system by activating macrophages, the white blood cells that initiate the immune response. Interferon injections have been effective in treating leukemia and MS. Common side effects include nausea, diarrhea, headache, fever, and flu-like symptoms.

Immunoglobulin injections are commonly used to treat a variety of disorders, including immune deficiencies, serious infections, and autoimmune and inflammatory disorders. For example, it has been used to treat neuropathy, Guillain-Barré syndrome, Kawasaki disease, lupus erythematosus, juvenile arthritis, and MS. Side effects include headache, low-grade fever, chills, anemia, low-back pain, and nausea.

Nonsteroidal Anti-Inflammatory Drugs (NSAIDs)

NSAIDs—such as ibuprofen (Advil, Nuprin, and Motrin), naproxen (Aleve), or the newer COX-2 inhibitors (Celebrex, Vioxx)—are used for a wide variety of aches and pains. While inflammation is a normal part of the healing process, it can get out of hand—for example, in chronic rheumatoid arthritis—and inflammation itself can become a disease. NSAIDs such as ibuprofen and naproxen ameliorate pain and other symptoms associated with inflammation. Technically speaking, NSAIDs decrease circulating lymphocytes and monocytes, lymphocyte activity, antibody and complement levels, inflammation, and general immunity. In very basic terms, they suppress an overactive immune system.

While NSAIDs are generally safe if taken once a week or less, it's estimated that more than 16,500 people die from, and more than 100,000 are hospitalized for, NSAID side effects.[29] The most common NSAID side effects involve the digestive tract, including nausea, gas, stomach ulcers, and gastrointestinal bleeding. To reduce gastrointestinal symptoms, take NSAIDs with food or milk. Other side effects include headaches, high blood pressure, dizziness, drowsiness, and ringing in the ears. Long-term use or high doses can cause liver and kidney damage. Talk to your doctor before using NSAIDs if you are allergic to aspirin, pregnant, or breast-feeding, or if you have a peptic ulcer or a history of gastrointestinal bleeding, kidney, liver, or heart disease, uncontrolled high blood pressure, anemia, or autoimmune disease. Don't take NSAIDs if you are taking blood thinners (anticoagulants), corticosteroids (such as prednisone), lithium, or oral anti-diabetic medications.[30]

The newer COX-2 inhibitors offer relief to people who can't tolerate NSAID digestive side effects. While most NSAIDs work by suppressing two types of the cyclooxygenase enzyme—COX-1 and COX-2—COX-2 inhibitors suppress only COX-2, the type associated with inflammation. The COX-1 enzyme is thought to protect the stomach lining, and disabling the enzyme is thought to cause side effects such as stomach bleeding, stomach ulcers, and kidney and liver problems. However, pharmaceutical maker Merck recalled Vioxx in September 2004 when a study showed an increased risk for heart attack and stroke among people taking it for 18 months or more.[31] It appears that other NSAIDs can also increase the risk of heart attack and stroke.

Narcotic Analgesics

Narcotic analgesics, commonly prescribed for chronic pain and cancer, include opium derivatives or opiates, such as codeine, morphine, and heroin, and opioids, which are synthesized to produce the same effect as opium. It's thought that opiates work by mimicking our own natural endorphins, whose job is to regulate the transmission of pain from the peripheral nervous system to the central nervous system.

Narcotic analgesics are restricted because of their addictive character, and are often either overused or underused. The right amount can give patients welcome relief, but too much can be harmful, and too little doesn't help. Because of the likelihood of dependence with prolonged use, if you are still in pain on narcotics, it's worth talking with your doctor about increasing the dose, or discontinuing the drug and trying a less addictive drug, or trying complementary therapies like herbs or acupuncture. Commonly used narcotic drugs include Demerol, Vicodin, Percodan, Percocet, OxyContin, Fentanyl, Dilaudid, and Duragesic (Fentanyl delivered via a transdermal patch).

Sleep Aids

Old-style barbiturate sleeping pills have largely been replaced by newer nonbarbiturate drugs, such as zolpidem (Ambien), that aren't addictive and have more limited side effects. Prolonged use of barbiturates causes tolerance and physical dependence. Barbiturates are the drugs most frequently used in suicide. Benzodiazepine sleep aids are slower to cause tolerance and less likely to cause physical dependence than barbiturates, and include flurazepam (Dalmane), estazolam (ProSom), quazepam (Doral), and temazepam (Restoril). Sleep aids available without a prescription include diphenhydramine (Nytol, Sleep-Eze, and Sominex) and doxylamine (in Unisom Nighttime), which contain a sedating antihistamine that can cause daytime drowsiness. People also commonly use over-the-counter antihistamines to help them sleep, but these medications have unpleasant side effects including dry mouth or mucous membranes, drowsiness, headache, vertigo, dizziness, insomnia, jitteriness, nausea, and diarrhea. For ideas on how to improve your sleep without drugs, see the "Insomnia" section of Chapter Three.

Steroids (Corticosteroids, Prednisone, Prednisolone)

Corticosteroids are hormones secreted in the adrenal cortex, the outer part of the small adrenal glands found at the top of each kidney. Because they suppress the immune system, steroid drugs such as prednisone and prednisolone are often prescribed for patients diagnosed with asthma, rheumatoid arthritis, lupus, multiple sclerosis (MS), and inflammatory bowel disease (Crohn's disease and ulcerative colitis). In the short term, steroids reduce inflammation and stop an overactive immune response. However, the side effects of high-dose or long-term use of steroids can be serious, including "moon face," weight gain, increased infections, decreased bone density, high blood pressure, diabetes, cataracts and glaucoma, male infertility, and loss of muscle mass. Additional side effects include abdominal pain, skin problems, irregular heartbeat, muscle cramps, fatigue, bodily pain or weakness, nausea and vomiting, thin skin, bruising easily, wounds that won't heal, eye disorders, osteoporosis, euphoria, depression, insomnia, nosebleeds, increased facial or body hair, facial flushing, and anxiety.

While you are taking steroids, your physician should monitor your glucose levels, hypothalamus and pituitary function, and potassium, sodium, and calcium levels, as well as perform regular eye exams. Corticosteroid dosages should be decreased gradually under the supervision of your health professional—abrupt withdrawal from long-term steroid use can cause severe depression. Licorice and other herbs can make the steroid withdrawal process smoother. Please see a professional herbalist.

Chapter Two

Immune Herbs and Nutrients

Herbs and supplements can give patients control over their health. Patients who feel like they have some control over their bodies always do better than patients who are passive. Herbs are generally safer, are slower acting, and possess fewer side effects than drugs. In some cases they can be more effective, such as some viral infections, drug-resistant bacterial conditions, and many digestive and gynecological complaints. Herbs are often used alongside standard care for conditions such as infertility, cancer, and HIV. Herbal medicine can also be used to offset the side effects of biomedical treatments such as chemotherapy.

In many patients diagnosed with immune or autoimmune conditions, herbal therapies can bring the immune system back into balance. Appropriately used tonic herbs can boost vitality and protect against infection. Anti-toxin herbs treat viral and bacterial conditions, while others have anti-fungal and anti-parasitic effects. Herbs can be used to increase blood circulation and alleviate pain.

A hallmark of Chinese herbal medicine is that it uses combinations of four to twenty herbs in a tea or tablet form. In contrast, Western herbalists usually use fewer combinations of herbs.

One benefit of Chinese herbal medicine is that the practitioner pays special attention to the individual's constitution, or root health. The constitution can be determined by taking the patient's history, along with looking at the tongue and feeling the pulse. For example, an elderly woman recovering from chemotherapy is treated much differently if she comes down with a cold or flu, than a strapping young athlete who has similar symptoms.

Chinese herbs are prescribed to balance a patient's condition. If the patient feels hot and is running a temperature, the herbalist selects cooling herbs. In contrast, if the client feels cold and needs to put on sweaters when everyone in the house is in T-shirts, warming herbs are selected. The herbalist must always keep in mind the strength of the patient's overall health relative to the severity of the illness.

An herbalist must make an accurate diagnosis, select the most appropriate herb or formula for the individual, and select the correct method of administration and preparation. Because this process is complex, we recommend seeing a trained herbalist whenever possible. A qualified herbalist should make sure that the herbs they use are safe and effective. They should be able to make suggestions about how to combine herbs and supplements with any medication you are taking. Most herbalists keep their own pharmacy as they are trained in herbal quality control issues, whereas store personnel are usually not. Questions you might ask your herbalist include: What is your training? How much experience do you have using herbs in your practice? Have you ever treated a condition like mine? How long will it take before I get a response? The best way to find an herbalist is word of mouth. If you are not able to get a referral from a friend, family member, or other health professional, you can write to me at the address

116

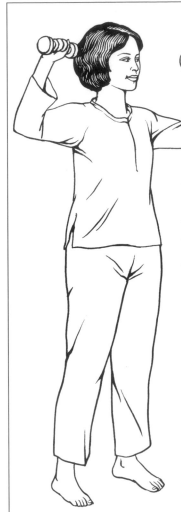

Shoulder Press

Stand with your legs shoulder width apart. Hold a weight in each hand at shoulder level, with your elbows bent and lose to your sides. Your palms should face inward. Slowly press the weights directly upward , until you arms are fully extended, and then bring them toward each other, allowing the end to touch directly over your heat. Don't rotate your wrists. Pause, and then separate you hands and slowly lower the weights to your shoulder. Do 12–15 repetitions per set, complete three sets.

About the Exercise Program in This Book

This program will strengthen your shoulder, arm, back, thigh, calf, and abdominal muscles. If you are not in shape you might consider starting with soup cans or three-pound weights, and gradually increase over time. There are a total of six exercises mentioned throughout the text. You might rest a minute or more after each set. Be sure to see your health professional before starting any exercise program.

in the Resource Guide in the appendices for the name of a professional who uses herbs in your area.

Herb Precautions

Purchase all your herbs from your herbalist; this way you can make sure the herbs you're taking are compatible with each other, and with any medications or supplements you are taking. Just as it's safer to get all your medications at the same pharmacy, where a professional can keep an eye on potential drug interactions, it's a good idea to get all your herbs from a professional herbalist who can make sure the herbs you are taking are compatible. Always keep your herbalist informed about the herbs and medications you are taking. Although they are much safer than drugs, herbs can interact with supplements, drugs, and foods. In our clinic, we have had clients get one herbal product from a neighbor, another from a health food store, and yet another from the Internet. This is far from ideal as quality may vary and there may be duplication and incompatibility.

In addition to consulting with an herbalist whenever possible, I also suggest using only herbal products manufactured in the U.S. Many raw herbs come from countries where regulations aren't as strict as they are in the U.S. with regards to cleanliness, purity requirements, and truth in labeling. In China and other countries, manufacturers aren't required to list product ingredients on the label, so products made in other countries often contain pharmaceutical drugs that are not disclosed on the label. In addition, sweeteners, allergens, and artificial colors and dyes are more likely to be found in foreign-made products.

Herbs and supplements should be used with great caution during pregnancy and nursing. Consult an herbalist. Although many herbs are safe during pregnancy, very few have been subject to clinical studies, and some are contraindicated during pregnancy. Until more is known, it's best to avoid using herbs during pregnancy. Follow your practitioner's suggestions and label directions carefully. Taking too little of an herb or supplement can produce no benefit, and taking too much can result in side effects such as a digestive reaction or a skin rash.

Children can use herbs, although if the child is under five we would always suggest seeing a trained professional. Children are usually dosed according to weight. Most product dosages are designed for 100- to 200-pound adults; therefore, for a child who weighs 30 pounds, one-third the adult dosage would be appropriate.

Herbs are far safer to use than drugs, and even conventional foods. Seeing a practitioner whenever possible, following directions carefully, and avoiding imported products can ensure you the best possible results. The next section discusses commonly used herbs and supplements, as well as ancient and modern formulas used in immune conditions.

Herbal Terms and Directions

Decoction—A decoction is tea made by simmering roots, bark, and stems typically for twenty minutes or longer. For whole herbs use approximately 1 oz. (30 g.) of herbs per 16 oz. of boiling water; strain before drinking.

Chinese Herbs—Take as directed by your herbalist.

Herbs in Tea Bags—Steep in teapot or a cup with a lid on for five to ten minutes.

Powdered Herbs—Simmer for two to three minutes and then cover and steep for ten to fifteen minutes and strain. Use 1 tsp. of powder to 8 oz. of boiling water.

Infusion (dried, cut, and sifted herbs)—Flowers, leaves, and thin stemmed herbs are steeped with a lid on for ten to fifteen minutes. Use 1–3 tsp. of herbs (depending upon weight) per cup of boiling water. Strain.

Poultice—A poultice is made by adding a small amount of hot or room temperature water to powdered herbs so they are damp. Apply the water/herb mixture to the skin (one-quarter-inch thick) and cover with breathable surgical tape or gauze. (Your herbalist may suggest adding aloe gel for burns and rejuvenation; honey, a natural antiseptic; healing oils; or liniments to the herbs.) To keep the poultice warm, wrap a heated water bottle or heating pad in cloth and apply over the poultice. If the poultice irritates the skin stop using. It's important to change the poultice at least once per day.

Fomentation (wash)—A cloth soaked in warm herbal decoction or infusion, strained and applied topically over the skin.

Tinctures—Tinctures are liquid alcohol herbal extracts that can be applied topically to the skin as directed by a health professional or internally as directed.

Salves—Salves can be made by simmering 3–4 tsp. of herb in oil (typically olive, safflower, or sesame) for one hour. Adding beeswax (4 Tbsp. per cup) may thicken it if added to warm herbal oil. Stir while the salve cools and thickens. More beeswax can be added if desired.

Bath—Two to four quarts of decoction and/or fifteen drops of essential oil can be added to an already drawn bath. Or add fresh chopped herbs or dried herbs wrapped in cheesecloth as the bath is filling up.

Soak—A soak is made by bathing an affected area in a decoction or infusion. Soaks are particularly useful for bruises, sprains, insect bites, and rashes.

Tablets and **Capsules** are the easiest way to take herbs. Typically herbs must be taken at higher dosages than drugs, so it is very important to take this dosage if you want to get the best results. Some herbalists recommend combining two or more formulas to customize your herbal blend. If you are self-treating, you may want to use one herb at a time.

Specific Remedies
Aloe

Aloe is used mainly for skin irritations and gastrointestinal complaints, and its polysaccharide components have anti-viral, anti-bacterial, anti-fungal, and immune-enhancing properties. Injections of acemannan—one of aloe's best-studied polysaccharides—are currently a drug approved for feline leukemia. Acemannan has also been shown to enhance T cell and interferon function. For example, in a study of fourteen HIV patients, taking 800 mg. of oral acemannan produced significant increases in circulating monocytes and macrophages. Follow-up studies showed an increase in T4, T8, and T24 antigen levels. Animal research has shown promising results in sarcomas and spontaneous tumors.[1]

Andrographis (*Andrographis paniculata*, chuan xin lian)

Andrographis is used widely both in China and in India, where it is known as *kalmegh*. It is traditionally used to treat infections, pharyngitis, laryngitis, pneumonia, herpes, skin infections, and snakebite. In Scandinavia, it is used to treat the common cold.

Studies in the U.S. and abroad have shown that andrographis boosts white blood cell and interferon production.[2] In Sweden, a controlled, double-blind study of fifty patients investigated the effectiveness of andrographis extracts in treating the flu. At a dosage of 1,200 mg. a day, 68 percent of the experimental group completely recovered after four days, versus 36 percent of the placebo group. Subjects using andrographis showed less fatigue, chills, sore throat, muscle aches, rhinitis, sinus pain, and headache than those using the placebo.[3] In a Chinese study of 131 pneumonia and chronic bronchitis patients, 79 percent showed an improvement in two weeks. In another Chinese clinical trial with 455 subjects, andrographis was considered 90 percent effective in treating childhood pneumonia, with an average of 3.1 days for fever to be normalized.

According to traditional Chinese medicine (TCM) theory, andrographis is used for clearing toxic heat, so it's cooling and shouldn't be used by patients with loose stools or cold signs such as low body temperature, cold extremities, and pallor. It may cause stomach pain in some individuals—if it does, the herb should be discontinued, or the dose decreased.

Artemisia (*Artemisia annua*, qing hao)

Artemisia has been used traditionally in the treatment of parasites and other unfriendly microbes. It has long been used in Chinese medicine to treat parasites, as a remedy for fevers, and particularly for malaria. A derivative of artemisia called artemisinin is a drug widely used to treat malaria; studies have found artemisinin to be an immunomodulator also effective in treating lupus and psoriasis. Artemisia has been used clinically to treat cancer, and has demonstrated anti-cancer activity on select cancer cells cultured in the laboratory.[4]

Astragalus (*Astragalus membranaceus*, huang qi)

Astragalus *(huang qi)* is traditionally used to improve the body's defensive energy, known in Chinese as *wei qi*. Astragalus is found in ancient herbal prescriptions for recovering strength following illness or exertion, fatigue, excessive perspiration, underweight, organ prolapse, and for healing burns. In the U.S. and China, astragalus is commonly used to help people with a variety of viral syndromes including HIV disease, herpes, chronic fatigue syndrome, and chronic hepatitis, and to bolster patients undergoing Western treatments for cancer. Of course, it should not be seen as a treatment for cancer, but rather as an adjunct to standard care.

Concern has been raised that astragalus may stimulate the immune system too much in autoimmune cases, but that hasn't been observed in American clinics specializing in traditional Chinese medicine (TCM). However, according to TCM theory, astragalus should not be used to treat a cold or flu because it might "tonify" the cold and make it worse, and should be used cautiously for individuals with digestive disorders because it can be difficult to digest.

Astragalus contains polysaccharides and flavones (isoflavone and quercetin) and saponins. Studies have shown it to have antioxidant, anti-bacterial, and anti-retroviral effects. Most of the modern research on astragalus has focused on its immune-enhancing effects. Laboratory studies have found astragalus to increase macrophages, T cell transformation, NK cell activity, interferon production, and phagocytosis. Astragalus seems to offer a preventive effect against the common cold, as reported in a Chinese study of 1,000 patients, in which subjects noticed fewer and shorter colds. The study also documented increased levels of IgA and IgG antibodies in nasal secretions after two months of treatment.[5] In another study, breast cancer patients given a combination of astragalus and ligustrum *(nu zhen zi)*—as an adjunct to radiation treatment—showed a decrease in death rate. In a study of patients undergoing chemotherapy for advanced lung cancer, mean survival time increased from 204 to 465 days for patients diagnosed with squamous cell carcinoma who were also taking astragalus, and from 192 to 324 days for patients with adenocarcinoma, compared with the group who received only chemotherapy.[6] Components of astragalus have been shown to reduce the immunosuppressive effects of the chemotherapy drug cyclophos-phamide.[7] Animal studies have also demonstrated that astragalus protects the liver.[8]

According to the Chinese pharmacopoeia, astragalus is graded and may be minimally processed or baked with honey. It is usually combined with other herbs in soups, teas, and pills.

Bupleurum (*Bupleurum chinense*, chai hu)

Bupleurum is an important ingredient in a long list of traditional Chinese formulas going back at least 1,800 years, and today it is one of the most popular herbs in Japan. Traditionally used to treat the liver, bupleurum formulas are also used to reduce fever and destroy viruses. In a study of 143 patients, those treated with bupleurum showed normalization of fever in 98.1 percent of influenza and 87.9 percent of common cold patients. When components of bupleurum were tested in the laboratory, results show anti-inflammatory, immune-modulating, and liver-protecting activity.[9]

While bupleurum is a safe herb, some precautions are necessary. It should always be taken under the guidance of a trained herbalist, as part of a formula, not as a single herb. Generally, bupleurum should not be used with headache, hypertension, or dry cough. It also should not be used with interferon, because a few cases of interstitial pneumonia have developed in patients using Minor Bupleurum Decoction (*xiao chai hu tang*) in conjunction with interferon treatments.

Citrus

Citrus peel is commonly used in traditional Chinese formulas to aid and smooth digestion. Modified citrus pectin and limonene are two contemporary citrus-derived supplements that are currently getting researchers' attention for their cancer-fighting potential.

Modified citrus pectin supplements have been shown to improve PSA (prostate-specific antigen) levels in two human small-scale studies. In animal studies, it has been shown to shrink colon cancer tumors, prevent breast cancer from spreading, and decrease melanoma metastasis.[10] Modified citrus pectin is a form of fruit fiber, like the apple pectin used to make jam, in which the molecules have been broken down into smaller molecules so that they can move across the intestinal lining and into the bloodstream.[11] Modified citrus pectin seems to prevent cancer growth by surrounding the galectins on the surface of cells. Galectins help cells connect to each other, and cancer cells have more galectins than normal cells, which allow them to spread the cancer.[12]

Limonene is a substance found in the peel of citrus fruits, and is being tested for actions against cancer. It is thought to block proteins that stimulate cell growth and reproduction, thus protecting against cancer, shrinking tumors, and slowing tumor growth. A concentrated form of limonene has been found to shrink breast cancers in animals.[13]

Codonopsis (*Codonopsis pilosula*, dang shen)

Codonopsis is typically administered as a less expensive, milder substitute for Asian ginseng. It contains volatile oils, polysaccharides, insulin, saponins, glucosides, and resins. While its uses are similar to those of Asian ginseng, many practitioners consider it better than Asian ginseng for building the blood. Laboratory experiments have shown that codonopsis may enhance phagocytosis of the reticuloendothelial system, thus improving immune system function. Research has also demonstrated that codonopsis increases respiratory rate, and red blood cell and hemoglobin counts.[14]

Coptis (*Coptis chinensis*, huang lian)

Coptis is a dark yellow herb that contains berberine, among several alkaloids. Coptis is considered one of the strongest antibacterial herbs and is used in the treatment of dysentery, gastroenteritis, cholera, respiratory tract infections, ear, nose, and throat infections, mouth sores, and skin infections. Due to its bitter taste, it is usually administered in tablet or capsule form.

Cordyceps (*Cordyceps sinensis*, dong chong xia cao)

Cordyceps, also known as caterpillar fungus, is a tonic herb known for its ability to increase vitality, clear the lungs, and improve endurance. In Chinese medicine terms, cordyceps is said to nourish the kidney yin and yang and to protect the lungs. Today, cordyceps is used to treat respiratory conditions, to support patients undergoing chemotherapy and radiation treatment, and to treat impotence, as well as hepatitis, kidney failure, diabetes, and chronic fatigue. Cordyceps has also been used to help people recover from debilitating illness, and to boost athletes' performance.

Research shows that cordyceps contains L-tryptophan and other amino acids. It stimulates interferon activity, inhibits bacteria and hepatitis B virus, enhances the function of the adrenal cortex, increases respiratory muscle performance, and calms the nervous system by balancing the hypothalamus/pituitary axis. It also increases the production of ATP, the body's energy storehouse molecule, by as much as 50 percent. Cardiovascular benefits include increased cardiac output and decreased platelet aggregation. Cordyceps is used in Chinese hospitals and clinics for chronic bronchitis, asthma, congestive heart disease, and tuberculosis and other respiratory conditions, and to improve a patient's tolerance for chemotherapy and radiation. Studies in China have shown that patients taking cordyceps have less coughing and wheezing, have fewer asthmatic symptoms, and catch fewer colds. Studies at Cornell University in New York found that cordyceps extract counteracted the effects of immune-suppressing chemotherapy drugs on T-helper cells, decreasing pain and fatigue, and in some cases, shrinking tumors.

Cordyceps is traditionally taken both as a tonic food and as medicine. It may be prepared with chicken, duck, or pork, boiled as a tea, or taken in pill form. Be careful with raw cordyceps packets found in Chinatown; lead has been inserted into the picked fungus before drying to bulk up the weight. It's best to buy dry extract from suppliers specializing in Chinese medicine. The general dosage is 1 to 3 g. of extract per day. For maximum absorption, it should be taken on an empty stomach, but if intestinal gas or bloating is observed, take it with meals. General response time is two to six weeks.

Coriolus (*Coriolus versicolor*, yun zhi)

Coriolus is a mushroom commonly called the "turkey tail" in North America for its brown and gray variegated coloring. In Chinese medicine, coriolus is used to dispel dampness, reduce phlegm, treat pulmonary infections, and support liver health. Coriolus is extremely popular in China and Japan. In fact, in Japan, the government approved its coverage by health insurance, and it is used extensively there for people receiving chemotherapy and radiation.

More than 400 clinical studies have demonstrated that coriolus polysaccharide extracts have immune-modulating and anti-tumor effects. When given as an adjuvant during conventional therapy for cancer, coriolus has significantly increased survival rates. Japanese research shows that coriolus extract has anti-tumor effects and stimulates natural killer (NK) cells. Used in conjunction with chemo and radiation therapy, coriolus has been found to be instrumental in helping increase cancer survival rates. Coriolus also stimulates the production of killer T cells and tumor necrosis factor (TNF), and activates macrophage function. Coriolus is also used as an adjunct for hepatitis and lung infections.

In a study published in *Lancet,* a group of 262 gastric cancer patients who underwent gastrectomy followed by chemotherapy were randomly divided into two groups. The group that was placed on coriolus during chemotherapy had a survival rate of 73 percent as opposed to 60 percent for the group that underwent chemotherapy alone.[15] Another study was conducted with 185 patients with stages I, II, or III non-small cell lung cancer who were treated with radiotherapy. Those with stages I or II who were administered coriolus had a 39 percent five-year survival rate as opposed to the 22 percent and 16 percent survival rates, respectively, of patients of the same disease stages who had not received coriolus. Stage III patients who took coriolus had a 22 percent survival rate versus none for the non-coriolus group.[16]

Cancers reported to respond to coriolus include stomach, uterine, colon, lung, colorectal, prostate, breast, and liver. In the overall treatment of cancer, coriolus seems to be most beneficial when used as an adjunct to conventional therapeutic regimens. Researchers suggest that coriolus appears to counteract the immune suppression of the conventional therapies and the toxic processes of cancer proliferation. Ongoing research shows that coriolus also has anti-viral activity, and appears to be effective against HIV infection. Additionally, animal studies indicate that coriolus seems to have cholesterol-lowering effects, as well as diuretic and mild tranquilizing effects.

Deer antler (*Cornu cervi parvum (pharmaceutical) or Cervus nippon (zoological)*, lu rong)

Deer antler—along with its extracts, such as pantocrine—is considered one of the strongest tonic herbs, and is particularly good for seniors. It is traditionally used to increase strength, build blood, heal fractures, and eliminate pain. Laboratory experiments have demonstrated that deer antler and its extracts increase oxygen uptake, increase red and white blood cells, and promote the healing of wounds and fractures.

Antler dosage should always start low, increasing over time if tolerance is good. In Chinese medicine, deer antler is considered to be very warming, and too much can cause increased body temperature, headache, bleeding, and digestive disorders. Antler is contraindicated for patients who have heat signs such as elevated body temperature, afternoon fevers, or feeling warm when others are not. Some practitioners consider antler to be contraindicated for children and adolescents. Use under professional supervision. Because it is so expensive and prone to spoilage, deer antler is usually taken as a pill or alcohol extract.

Echinacea (purple coneflower, *Echinacea angustifolia/purpurea/pallida*)

Echinacea is considered to be an immune stimulant because it increases the body's ability to destroy bacteria and viruses. In more than 200 scientific studies, echinacea has been demonstrated to have anti-bacterial, anti-viral, and anti-inflammatory effects. Three species of echinacea are in common use. *Angustifolia* was the most widely used in the U.S. until the 1980s, when *purpurea* became more popular because it is easier to cultivate; therefore, most of the research has been conducted with *purpurea*. *Pallida* is mostly used as a cheaper substitute for the other species.

In a double-blind, placebo-controlled study, *Echinacea purpurea* was administered to 180 patients, comparing two different dosages. Subjects taking 900 mg. per day had statistically significant improvement in symptoms such as stuffy nose, sneezing, sore throat, and headache, as compared to the placebo group. Interestingly, patients taking 450 mg. of echinacea did not show a significant improvement.[17] Echinacea comes in many forms: solid, extract, tincture, tea, juice, and powder. Echinacea is available by itself, and also with other herbs for broad-spectrum effects. Traditionally, echinacea was not recommended for long-term use.

Eclipta (*Eclipta prostrata*, han lian cao)

In Chinese medicine, eclipta has traditionally been thought to nourish the liver and kidney yin, and to cool the blood to stop bleeding. It has been used to treat tinnitus, premature graying of the hair, and various kinds of bleeding. In the Ayurvedic system of medicine, preparations of eclipta are used to treat cirrhosis of the liver. According to modern research, an ethyl acetate of eclipta gave even better protection than silymarin one of the active components in milk thistle, in liver cells exposed to toxins. Leading pharmacological researcher Hildebert Wagner of Germany considers eclipta to be one of the most promising liver protective herbs.[18]

Eleuthero root *(Eleutherococcus senticosus,* ci wu jia)

Eleuthero root is a distant relative of true ginseng, and considered by traditional herbalists to be much weaker than either Asian or American ginseng. It is most extensively used and researched in Russia, where it is used to help the body adapt to stress and is given to astronauts, athletes, and rescue workers to increase performance. Since 1962, 6,000 patients have been involved in clinical trials in which eleuthero was found to improve mental alertness and work quality with minimal side effects.[19]

Forsythia *(Forsythia suspensa,* lian qiao)

Known for its bright yellow flowers, forsythia is traditionally used in formulas that detoxify and dispel heat, including *Yin Chao,* a popular Chinese cold remedy. Modern laboratory studies have found forsythia to offer broad-spectrum anti-bacterial effects. It is often used today in formulas for fever, sore throat, carbuncles and other inflammatory skin conditions, swollen lymph nodes, and urinary tract infections. In one case study, eight patients with acute nephritis all experienced reduced edema and blood pressure after taking forsythia as a decoction three times per day before meals.[20]

131

Garlic

Garlic is used throughout the world for its anti-microbial properties, and in Asia, it's been used medicinally for several thousand years. And for good reason—garlic offers a broad-spectrum effect against bacteria, viruses, fungus, and parasites. Garlic inhibits a long list of bacteria including staphylococcus aureus (staph), streptococcus (strep), E. coli, salmonella, citrobacter, klebsiella pneumoniae, and mycobacteria. It also fights fungus, including candida. In addition, garlic kills common and troublesome viruses such as herpes simplex 1 and 2 virus, rhinovirus, vaccinia virus, and vesicular stomatitis. In China, it's been observed that there is less cancer among the populations that consume the most garlic.

The best way to use garlic for its anti-microbial qualities is to crush a whole clove, let it sit for ten to twenty minutes, then add to homemade yogurt or mix with pure water before consuming. In terms of TCM, garlic is considered warming and should be used only with caution if heat signs are present. Furthermore, some clients have digestive intolerance to garlic. General therapeutic dosage is one to three cloves per day.

Ginseng (Panax, American, eleuthero, codonopsis)

The three popularly used species of ginseng are Asian ginseng (also called *panax ginseng,* ren shen), American ginseng *(panax quinquefolium,* xi yang shen), and tienchi *(notoginseng,* san qi). Common substitutes for ginseng include eleuthero, also known as Siberian ginseng *(eleutherococcus senticosus,* ci wu jia), and codonopsis (dang shen).

American Ginseng
(*Panax quinquefolium l.*, xi yang shen)

American ginseng typically grows on the east coast of Canada and the U.S. It has an anti-stress effect similar to that of Asian ginseng, with several important differences. First, while Asian ginseng is considered warming in TCM, American ginseng is cooling, and so more suitable for patients who are physically robust, and have symptoms like afternoon fevers, dry cough, and digestive disorders. It is usually more appropriate for children because they're generally more active, yang, and warm. It's also more effective for diabetes. American ginseng's mild taste makes for a better beverage than Asian ginseng, but vials and pre-made teas containing any form of ginseng may also contain a lot of sugar, honey, or even artificial sweeteners, which is why I don't suggest "instant" forms of ginseng. In Chinese hospitals, patients drink American ginseng infused in hot water throughout the day, along with their other herbal decoctions.

Asian Ginseng (*Panax ginseng,* ren shen)

Asian ginseng has a special place in the Chinese pharmacopoeia. The name *panax* is derived from the Greek word for "all healing," as in *panacea.* Asian ginseng has special properties for rescuing the dying by preventing heart collapse, tranquilizing the spirit, and generating fluids. In TCM, Asian ginseng is a general tonic for "invigorating the primal qi," and is used in many ancient prescriptions for a multitude of conditions. Ginseng is not, however, by itself, good for the same multitude of conditions, and this creates a misunderstanding. Asian ginseng's benefits vary depending on the herbs it's combined with. Asian ginseng is particularly good for people of advanced age or in a debilitated state.

133

It is used in formulas for general weakness, fatigue, anemia, diabetes, chronic fatigue syndrome, fibromyalgia, impotence, and infertility.

Wild ginseng is most revered, and it is exceptionally expensive, easily running several thousand dollars for a few grams. Even cultivated ginseng can cost several thousand dollars per pound. There are various grades of ginseng, depending on the growing region, as well as the size and appearance of the root. Traditionally, only the roots were used, but scientific experiments have shown that leaves, flowers, and stems all have medicinal value, but because not much is known about their use, they are not recommended for general consumption. A further distinction is made depending upon how the ginseng is prepared. For example, white ginseng is prepared simply by drying the roots after removing the outer layer, and is considered neutral and moistening. Red ginseng is made by steaming the root, giving it a reddish brown appearance, and is considered warming. Tienchi (panax notoginseng), a relative of ginseng called *san qi* in Chinese medicine, is primarily used to increase blood circulation, especially in the treatment of injuries due to trauma, surgery, or cancer.

Asian ginseng enhances phagocytosis and nonspecific immunity. Experimental studies have demonstrated that ginseng helps the body adapt to stress, and can reactivate the pituitary and adrenal systems. In animal experiments, ginseng has been shown to stimulate protein synthesis, and to suppress the growth of cancer cells. Ginseng enhances phagocytosis of the reticuloendothelial system, increases erythrocytes, hemoglobin, and leukocytes, and protects against radiation damage.[21] A survey of more than 1,800 patients at a hospital in Seoul, Korea, found that people who consumed ginseng were less likely to have cancer. Animal studies show ginseng and some of its constituents inhibit the growth of ovarian cancer cells, lung tumors, and liver tumors.[22]

Asian ginseng contains trace amounts of vitamins, amino acids, enzymes, and saponin glycosides termed ginsenosides. At least thirty different ginsenosides have been identified by Chinese, Japanese, and Korean researchers. Although in the West one can find ginseng products advertised for their "ginsenoside" content, these products are rarely used by doctors of TCM, who prefer to make tea or concentrates of the whole plant. In fact, some of those ginsenoside products are made from the weaker leaf.

Asian ginseng is not traditionally used for children, unless they are exceptionally weak. It is contraindicated for excess conditions such as fever, irritability, facial flushing, nosebleeds, and digestive cramping and bloating. It is also not traditionally used for people with parasitic infections. Ginseng should not be used along with other stimulants, such as caffeine.

Goldenseal

Known as "king of the mucous membranes," goldenseal has been traditionally used as a wash for eye conditions, and as an antiseptic, astringent, and anti-inflammatory for the mouth, sinuses, throat, lungs, digestive tract, and skin. Goldenseal contains berberine, which has anti-bacterial, anti-fungal, and anti-parasitic effects. It is generally recommended that goldenseal be taken for short periods of time—for most cases, using goldenseal for longer than ten days is inappropriate. Dosage is 1,000–3,000 mg. per day. Contrary to popular belief, goldenseal does not mask the presence of illegal drugs.

Green Tea

Next to water, tea is the most popular beverage in the world, and for good reason, green tea has a long list of health benefits. Tea comes from camellia sinensis, a shrub native to Asia. Unlike black or oolong tea, green tea is not fermented, and so is cooler in nature, and better for people with inflammation or heat symptoms.

Tea is rich in powerful antioxidant flavonoids called catechins, which are very well absorbed by the body compared with other flavonoids. Catechins have been shown to inhibit certain cancers, improve blood flow in the cardiovascular system, and reduce LDL cholesterol oxidation. In addition, recent research has shown the catechins in green tea to be thermogenic, helping dieters shed fat, according to research published in the December 1999 issue of the *American Journal of Clinical Nutrition*. Other new research shows that green tea catechins are strong vasodilators, increasing blood flow.

Green tea may be good for diabetics, because it lowers serum glucose levels by inhibiting the starch-digesting enzyme amylase, so that starch is absorbed more slowly, and insulin levels decrease. Diphenylamine, a compound found in green tea, also seems to lower blood sugar. Green tea has been shown to lower intestinal fat absorption as well. Green tea also raises brain levels of serotonin and dopamine, which control both the appetite and satiety response, as well as mood.

Laboratory experiments have demonstrated that constituents of tea reduce the growth of cancer cells and the growth of certain tumors. A lowered incidence of stomach cancer has been observed in populations that drink green tea regularly. Additional studies suggest that green tea may also reduce the risk of colon and pancreatic cancer.[23] In a study of 8,552 Japanese men and women over the age of forty, the people who drank tea regularly had a lowered incidence of cancer.[24] In a seven-year study of 472 women with breast cancer, increased green tea consumption was associated with decreased numbers of lymph node metastases in pre-menopausal women with stage 1 and 2 breast cancer. Long-term consumption of more than five cups of tea daily was also significantly associated with decreased cancer recurrence in stage 1 and 2 patients who were in remission at the time of the follow-up study six years later. Green tea showed no effect in stage 3 breast cancer patients.[25]

Tea's anti-inflammatory effects are similar to those of COX-2 anti-inflammatory drugs. Black and green tea both deactivate viruses, metabolize fat, improve artery function, and inhibit cancer growth. According to researchers at Rutgers University, a compound in black tea called TF-2 caused colorectal cancer cells to "commit suicide." Normal cells were unaffected according to Rutgers researcher Kuang Yu Chen, Ph.D. Tea consumption has also been tied to a lower risk of stomach, colon, and breast cancer.[26] Tea contains theanine, an amino acid that may reduce the toxicity of chemotherapy. Theanine improves anti-tumor activity in bone marrow and in the liver, and protects against ovarian cancer.[27] In addition, tea helps prevent DNA damage to the skin and helps minimize UV effects, which could minimize the risk of skin cancer and aging.

How does tea work? Green tea has a constituent called polyphenols, which are potent antioxidants. Green tea's polyphenols appear to detoxify cancer-causing agents, suppress the activity of carcinogens, and inhibit the formation of cancer-causing compounds such as nitrosamines.[28] Lab studies show that green tea extracts inhibit the growth of breast cancer cells.[29]

Green tea is best taken in tea form to get the highest dose with minimal additives and processing. Three cups per day is an average suitable dose, in place of less helpful caffeine-containing beverages like coffee or soda. As with any caffeinated product, reduce the dosage if nervousness, anxiety, or insomnia occur.

Green tea polyphenols are also available in supplement form. Typical dosage is 200−500 mg. daily.

Isatis *(Isatis tinctoria,* da qing ye and ban lan gen)

The isatis plant is the source of indigo, and has two medicinal parts: the root, known as *ban lan gen* in Chinese, and the leaf, known as *da qing ye.* The root is more widely used in the U.S. Isatis is traditionally used to clear heat and fever, decrease inflammation, and detoxify. It is widely used for a variety of bacterial and viral infections including influenza, hepatitis, mononucleosis, and chronic fatigue syndrome. Isatis root contains indoxyl-beta-glucoside, indirubin, as well as resins and polysaccharides.

Laboratory studies have demonstrated isatis' anti-inflammatory, phagocyte-enhancing and fever-reducing properties, and its ability to inhibit a long list of pathogens, including: staphylococcus aureus, diplococcus pneumoniae, alpha streptococcus, haemophilus influenzae, E. (escherichia) coli, salmonella typhi, and shigella dysenteriae.

Clinical studies confirm isatis' healing properties. In one study of 326 cases of upper respiratory infection, the herb decoction was considered effective in all cases.[30] In the treatment of 300 cases of acute bacillary dysentery and gastroenteritis, fever subsided after one day of taking the decoction, and stool examination was normalized within five days.[31] In 43 cases of mononucleosis, subjective symptoms improved significantly in three to five days, along with a reduction in fever and a decrease in abnormal lymphocytes. According to researchers, isatis was more effective in young children than adults.[32] Isatis was also judged to be 76.4 percent effective in case reports on the treatment of viral skin conditions such as herpes simplex and herpes zoster.[33]

Isatis leaf contains similar constituents to the root, and acts against a similar list of pathogenic organisms in lab tests (see above). It is traditionally used for its heat-clearing, fever-reducing, and anti–inflammatory effects. Today it is used as a remedy for fever, pharyngolaryngitis, and carbuncles, as well as skin and digestive tract ulcerations. Isatis preparations are well tolerated, though they should not be used with low body temperature or subjective complaints of cold without fever, and should be used cautiously with diarrhea.

Licorice (*Glycyrrhiza uralensis*, gan cao)

Licorice is called "sweet root" by many cultures, and Chinese herbalists call it the "great harmonizer." Licorice is traditionally used in Chinese formulas as a harmonizing ingredient, and one that boosts spleen qi. In the West, licorice is primarily used as a sweetener and for treating ulcers. In regards to immunity, licorice has been shown to have anti-inflammatory, anti-tumor, anti-allergic, and liver-protecting effects. Licorice increases the production of interferon and NK cell activity.

Researchers in China and Japan consider the component glycyrrhizia to be central to licorice's immune-regulating effects. Laboratory reports have shown that licorice enhances phagocytic function, induces interferon, anti-allergic, anti-inflammatory, and possibly tumor-inhibiting effects. Licorice prolongs the action of cortisol[34] by stimulating the adrenal cortex. Licorice is thought to transform toxins in the liver into insoluble waste products, thus improving liver function. Chinese studies have demonstrated its ability to reduce liver pain and hepatomegaly in hepatitis patients.

Licorice may raise blood pressure in susceptible individuals, especially at doses of more than 5 g. per day. High doses of licorice have been shown to produce edema, headache, and upset of sodium/potassium levels. For these reasons, it is important to use licorice with supporting herbs to mitigate potential side effects. Professional guidance is recommended if you are consuming licorice by itself for longer than three months.

Ligustrum *(Ligustrum lucidum,* nu zhen zi)

Ligustrum is a small fruit that contains oleanolic acid and oxalic acid, along with other constituents including syringin, nueshenide, linolenic acid, palmitic acid, and oeuropenin. In Chinese medicine, ligustrum is known as a yin tonifying herb and is used in formulas for infertility, backache, dizziness, ringing in the ears, and blurred vision. Because it increases white blood cell production, ligustrum is used in China to prevent and treat leukopenia caused by chemotherapy and radiotherapy.[35] In a clinical evaluation at MD Anderson Hospital in Houston, Texas, ligustrum improved subjects' tolerance for chemotherapy and radiation. Ligustrum leaf has been studied in China to treat bronchitis.

Lonicera *(Lonicera japonica,* jin yin hua)

Known as honeysuckle in the U.S., lonicera's Chinese name *jin yin hua* translates as "gold and silver flower." Its anti-bacterial and anti-viral effects make lonicera one of the chief ingredients in *Yin Chao*—a well-known cold remedy—and it is widely found in herbal formulas used to treat colds, flus, upper respiratory infections, conjunctivitis, mastitis, tonsillitis, pneumonia, dysentery, appendicitis, fever, nasal infections, carbuncles, ulcerative colitis, hepatitis, and cervical infection. Lab experiments have shown lonicera to have a strong anti-bacterial effect against salmonella typhi, pseudomonas aeruginosa, staphylococcus aureus, and staphylococcus pneumoniae.

Lycium (*Lycium chinense*, gou qi zi)

Lycium is a bright red fruit that has traditionally been used by itself as a food, or with other herbs, as a longevity tonic. In Chinese medicine, it is used to nourish the blood, improve function of the eyes, and when combined with other kidney tonics, treat a variety of age-related conditions. In lab experiments, lycium polysaccharides enhanced macrophage, T- and B-lymphocytes, and NK cells.

Lycium tastes sweet, so it can be taken by itself, or combined with foods, or in decoctions or pills. It is generally well tolerated, though it may cause digestive symptoms in some patients. The bark of the lycium tree—*di gu pi* in Chinese—is used to reduce night sweats, inflammation, and heat.

Marijuana

Marijuana has been used since biblical times, though today it is illegal in many countries. Some states, including California, have passed medical marijuana laws that enable citizens to use marijuana for medical purposes without fear of arrest. As one experienced doctor attests, "Working with AIDS and cancer patients, I repeatedly saw how marijuana could ameliorate a patient's debilitating fatigue, restore appetite, diminish pain, remedy nausea, cure vomiting, and curtail down-to-the-bone weight loss." Synthetic THC, the active ingredient in marijuana, is available in the prescription drug dronabinol (Marinol), which is approved by the FDA to treat nausea and vomiting associated with chemotherapy, and to treat appetite loss and weight loss in people with AIDS. Many cancer and HIV patients, however, have found that smoked marijuana works faster and is more effective than the synthetic version. Smoked marijuana also allows the patient to control the dose.

Is marijuana a cure-all? No. While it may have promise as a medicine for people with AIDS, cancer, and chronic pain, most people with immune disorders should use it cautiously for a number of reasons. Laboratory experiments have shown that the component chemicals in marijuana reduce resistance to bacterial, protozoan, and viral infection. Cannabis plants may be contaminated by fungal spores, increasing the risk of fungal infection. Marijuana use can contribute to birth defects if used during pregnancy, change the balance between male and female sex hormones, reduce sperm counts, and cause irregular menstruation. It may also cause symptoms of anxiety including overreaction, apprehension, sweating, tremors, and shakes. Additionally, marijuana can increase the heart rate and disturb heart rhythms. Marijuana smokers predispose themselves to lung cancer, sinus problems, coughing, and sore throats. Smoking marijuana is associated with chronic bronchitis, coughing, phlegm production, shortness of breath, and wheezing, according to a study published in the *Journal of General Internal Medicine*,[36] which based its results on 6,728 questionnaires completed by adults twenty to fifty-nine years of age.

Marijuana may also increase susceptibility to infection and disable the immune system. Other side effects of marijuana use include impaired coordination, judgment, and short-term memory, mood swings and irritability due to low blood sugar reactions, and blunted emotional development, especially in teenagers and preteens, which leads to coping problems. It is estimated that two million adult Americans are heavy marijuana users.

How does it work? Marijuana produces mild euphoria by releasing dopamine. It typically lasts longer than alcohol. Marijuana is much stronger now than it was in the 1970s. Today's marijuana contains up to 14 percent of the active ingredient THC (tetrahydrocannabinol), compared to 2–4 percent in the past. This increase in potency produces a longer, stronger high, and also a greater chance for addiction. THC lodges in the fatty cell walls of the brain and lingers in the body longer than other drugs and alcohol. Some people who are dependent on marijuana go into withdrawal right away; others notice withdrawal as it gradually clears the body. In order to break a habit with any drug, it is important to look at the reasons you use it. Do you use it to relax, do you use it for pain relief, or does it give you more energy? While smoking marijuana occasionally may not be any more harmful than occasional alcohol use, if your use is daily or even weekly, or if certain activities are just not the same without marijuana, it makes sense to get treatment. Further information can be found at www.marijuana-anonymous.org.[37]

Milk Thistle

Milk thistle has been used for hundreds of years to protect the liver, and also to increase breast milk. Silymarin, milk thistle's most important liver-protective constituent, has been shown to increase the glutathione content of the liver, which in turn increases the liver's detoxifying capacity. In addition, it has anti-inflammatory, antioxidant, and immune-modulating capabilities. Today milk thistle extracts, standardized to contain 80 percent silymarin, are used in Europe and North America to prevent liver damage and rebuild new liver cells. Milk thistle extract is also often recommended as a treatment for psoriasis.

In clinical studies, milk thistle extracts have produced clinical improvements in treating hepatitis, cirrhosis, and alcohol- and chemical-induced liver damage. In a study of 29 patients with viral hepatitis, those who took milk thistle showed decreased liver enzymes and bilirubin levels, when compared with a placebo group.[38] In a study of patients with chronic hepatitis, subjects taking 420 mg. of silymarin for three to twelve weeks experienced a reversal of liver cell damage and a decrease in liver enzymes. Subjects also reported improved appetite, digestive function, and energy levels.

Typical dosage is 140–160 mg. of silymarin three times daily, or three 200 mg. tablets containing 80 percent silymarin. Milk thistle extracts are generally safe for long-term use. If loose stools are noticed, decrease the dosage, and then increase it again when stools normalize.

Pau D'Arco (Lapachol)

Most popularly used as a treatment for intestinal and vaginal candida, Pau D'Arco is a South American herb that has traditionally been used to treat infections, digestive disorders, and skin disorders. In modern experiments, it has been found to have anti-bacterial, anti-viral, and anti-fungal properties. It has also been studied for its antineoplastic or tumor-reducing properties.

Take as a tea, two to eight cups a day. Boil 1 tsp. of Pau D'Arco for ten to fifteen minutes, and let it steep for ten minutes or longer. For vaginal candida, vaginitis, and cervicitis soak tampons in the decoction. Change at least every twenty-four hours, until the condition is resolved.

Phellodendron (*Phellodendron amurense or Phellodendron chinense*, huang bai)

Phellodendron contains berberine, which gives it its bright yellow color. Other plants containing berberine include goldenseal, coptis, and scute. Phellodendron is traditionally used for its heat-clearing effects. It is widely found in Chinese formulas for inflammatory conditions, skin infections, jaundice, fever, and hot flashes. Today in China, phellodendron is used in herbal formulas as a throat spray and in injectable forms.

In the laboratory, phellodendron has been found to inhibit many bacteria including staphylococcus aureus, streptococcus hemolyticus, E. coli, salmonella typhi, shigella, and mycobacterium tuberculosis. It also has an anti-fungal effect against trichomonas vaginalis, microsporum audouinii, and epidermophyton floccosum.

Reishi (*Ganoderma lucidum*, ling zhi)

Sometimes called the "mushroom for immortality," ganoderma has traditionally been used as a sedative and a Qi and blood tonic, and was used by monks to promote calmness, memory, and a meditative life, and to treat chest and heart conditions. Today, reishi is widely used to support the immune system in cancer patients, to protect the liver, to reduce cholesterol, blood glucose, and insomnia, and to treat hepatitis, bronchitis, cardiovascular disease, and autoimmune diseases including myasthenia gravis.

Clinical studies show reishi to improve symptoms of chronic bronchitis, and that it is particularly effective for cold and damp symptoms. It's also been shown to increase T-lymphocyte counts in patients with leukopenia caused by radiation and chemotherapy, and to lessen the side effects of these therapies.[39]

Under the microscope, ganoderma preparations promote regeneration of healthy liver cells and reduce inflammatory infiltration of hepatic lobules in mice. In the lab, ganoderma polysaccharides have been shown to increase lymphocytes both in normal spleen cells and in spleen cells suppressed by hydrocortisone. Lab experiments have also shown that ganoderma extract has anti-tumor properties, inhibiting a type of sarcoma and other tumor cells in mice. In the market there are two types of reishi, red and black. By far the most research has been done on the red reishi. We also recommend products made from the whole mushroom as opposed to the mycelium.

We don't recommend reishi tinctures because reishi is poorly soluble in alcohol, so tinctures don't give you an adequate dosage of active ingredients. Occasionally people get a rash from using reishi. If this occurs, stop taking it.

Rhubarb

Rhubarb is used as a laxative in both Chinese and Western herbology, but in TCM, it is also used to treat infection. Experimental studies show that rhubarb inhibits staphylococcus, streptococcus, typhoid, dysentery bacillus, and diphtheria bacillus. It also inhibits fungus, influenza virus, amebic dysentery, and trichomonas vaginalis.[40] In addition, rhubarb assists in removing endotoxins, the toxins created by harmful bacteria. According to Chinese experiments, rhubarb reduces platelet aggregation and bronchial spasm. Rhubarb is rarely taken by itself, and should be used as part of an herbal formula dispensed by a trained practitioner.

Schizandra (*Schizandra chinensis*, wu wei zi)

In Chinese, schizandra is known as *wu wei zi*—meaning "five-flavored fruit"—because it contains the five tastes of Chinese medicine: bitter, sweet, salty, sour, and pungent. In TCM, schizandra has been used as an astringent for the lungs and kidneys to reduce phlegm, sweating, incontinence, and coughing. It is traditionally used for nervous exhaustion, fatigue, insomnia, depression, diarrhea, and forgetfulness. Today, schizandra is considered to be an adaptogen that helps the body cope with stress, and is also used for its liver-protecting effects, especially in treating hepatitis.

Chinese studies including thousands of cases of hepatitis have shown specially processed schizandra to lower SGPT levels, and increase liver and glycogen synthesis.[41] One study noted that SGPT levels tended to rise six to twelve weeks after treatment was discontinued, which is why schizandra should not be discontinued suddenly, but rather, the dosage should be tapered off gradually. Animal studies have confirmed the liver-protecting effects of schizandra.[42]

Since the 1950s, Russian research has focused on schizandra's adaptogenic properties, which help the body adapt to stress, and its positive effects on mental and physical performance. For example, telegraph operators taking schizandra (5–10 mg./kg.) were found to increase productivity by 22 percent, with less fatigue.[43] In a study of 59 flight attendants taking schizandra, the experimental group did not notice an increase in heart rate or blood pressure while flying, as the controls did. And in a study of soldiers and athletes, "physical work capacity" was increased after twenty-one days of treatment, while it was unchanged in the placebo group.

To have an effect at reducing liver enzymes, schizandra must be specifically processed. For other indications, a standard preparation is suitable. Schizandra may aggravate peptic ulcers or stomach acidity, so it should be discontinued if this effect is noticed. It is also traditionally avoided in the early stages of colds, flu, and rashes, and not used with the Chinese herb *yu zhu* (polygonum odoratum).

Scute (*Scutellaria baicalensis*, huang qin)

Scute is found in several ancient Chinese herbal prescriptions, including *Xiao Chai Hu Tang*. It contains berberine, is considered bitter and cold, and is traditionally used in formulas for liver disorders, fever, cough, conjunctivitis, hypertension, and carbuncles. In laboratory experiments, scute has been shown to inhibit many viruses and to have anti-inflammatory broad-spectrum antibacterial, anti-allergy, diuretic, and fever-reducing effects. Baicalein, a constituent of scute, inhibits cancer cell multiplication.

Clinical studies in China have shown it to be useful in treating upper respiratory infections and bronchitis, and it has been used in Chinese hospitals to treat acute and chronic hepatitis, pancreatitis, and cholecystitis (gallbladder infection). Because scute is a cooling herb, it should be used cautiously with diarrhea and digestive conditions. A related herb, *Scutellaria barbata*, is used in Chinese clinics to treat cancer.

Shiitake

Shiitake is a medicinal and gourmet mushroom used for broad-spectrum immune support. In Japan, a shiitake extract called lentinan is used in injectable form. Shiitake appears to work by improving the body's immune response, instead of attacking tumors, viruses, or bacteria directly. Laboratory studies have shown

148

shiitake to increase natural killer (NK) cells; tumor necrosis factor, which helps fight tumors; and interleukin-1 and -2, which stimulate T cells.[44] Although shiitake extracts are available, I recommend consuming three to four large shiitake mushrooms daily in soup or tea form. Simmer for fifteen minutes—adding ginger and dates if desired for more flavor—then drink the broth and eat the mushrooms.

Smilax (*Smilax glabra,* tu fu ling)

Smilax is traditionally used to treat urinary tract infections, tumors, gout, and skin conditions. Smilax works by binding endotoxins, which aggravate the inflammatory process. In a study of 92 psoriasis patients, extracts of smilax greatly improved conditions in 62 percent of patients.[45] Despite attempts to market smilax as a natural testosterone supplement, there is no evidence that it is a sexual or bodybuilding aid.

Soy

Soy is high in isoflavones, a group of plant hormones, or phytoestrogens, similar to, though weaker than, human estrogen. Isoflavones offer a number of well-documented health benefits including reducing arterial plaque, thus reducing the risk for heart disease and stroke, reducing osteoporosis by stimulating bone formation, and relieving menopausal symptoms.

Commonly known for its usefulness in women's health issues including menopausal symptoms and osteoporosis, soy is currently being studied for its ability to prevent cancer, particularly prostate cancer. In an Australian study of 29 men with prostate cancer, patients who ate 2 oz. of soy grits a day saw a quick improvement in PSA (prostate-specific antigen) levels, which are used to screen for and to track prostate cancer.[46]

While soy has also been studied for its effect on breast cancer, these findings have been more mixed. High estrogen blood levels are associated with a higher risk for breast cancer, so by competing for space at estrogen receptors, the weaker soy isoflavones block the stronger human version, and thus lower estrogen blood levels. However, while some studies show isoflavones to have a protective effect against breast cancer, others suggest they may increase cancer risk.

St. John's Wort

Although chiefly known today as an herbal antidepressant, St. John's wort was traditionally used as a topical and internal remedy for nerve pain. In Europe, St. John's wort is a folk treatment for wounds, burns, and inflammation. St. John's wort contains hypericin, hyperiform, flavonoids, and essential oils. Lab studies have demonstrated the anti-viral effects of hypericin and pseudo-hypericin against herpes, influenza, and vesicular stomatitis virus.[47]

Look for a whole-herb, broad-spectrum extract that contains both hypericin and hyperiform. Typical dosage is 1 to 3 g. per day. Due to its cooling nature, St. John's wort can cause diarrhea and other digestive complaints. St. John's wort may also cause photosensitivity, so remember to wear sunscreen and a hat if you are outdoors while taking it.

Tang kuei (*Angelica sinensis*, dang gui)

Although known as a woman's herb in the U.S. because of its menstrual regulating effects, tang kuei is used in Chinese formulas

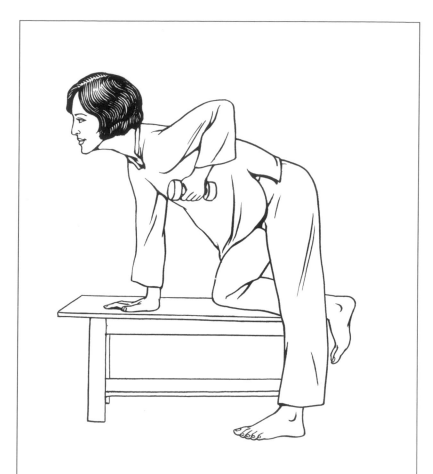

One Arm Row

Place your right hand and right knee on the bench (you can also use a low table or other object at knee height), and plant your left foot firmly on the floor next to the bench. Hold a weight in your left hand with your palm facing the left side of your body, and let your arm hang toward the floor. Bend your elbow, keeping it close to your body, and draw the weight toward your armpit as pictured. It is important to maintain a flat back. With the dumbbell near your armpit, pause, and then slowly lower your arm to the starting position. Do 12–15 repetitions per set; complete three sets on each side.

for immunity, respiratory, and circulatory conditions, as well as in trauma, anti-spasmodic, and pain-relieving formulas. It is traditionally used for its blood-building and circulation-improving properties.

Tang kuei contains vitamin B12, biotin, folic acid, and volatile oils. In laboratory studies, it has been used by itself and in traditional formulas such as *Si Wu Tang,* and has demonstrated non-specific immunological function.[48] Tang kuei and astragalus have proved useful in the treatment of immune pancytopenia and thrombocytopenic purpura. In one study, tang kuei tablets provided pain relief in twenty-three cases of herpes zoster. Ear acupoint injections of tang kuei have proved useful for skin diseases including hives, eczema, neurodermatitis, vitiligo, rosacea, and alopecia.

Tang kuei has a laxative effect, and may cause indigestion, especially if taken by itself. A literature review reveals that tang kuei does not have an estrogenic effect, although it has that reputation.

Viola (*Viola yedoensis,* zi hua di ding)

Viola was traditionally used in formulas for feverish conditions such as red eyes, painful throat, and mumps, and topically and internally for infections like carbuncles, boils, and breast abscess. It has also been used in both European and Chinese folk medicine as a cancer treatment. Viola has been shown to have anti-bacterial and anti-viral effects in laboratory experiments. For example, a 1988 study of twenty-seven herbs showed viola to have the strongest inhibitory effect against HIV in vitro. In Chinese medicine terms, viola clears heat, eliminates toxins, and relieves inflammation. Classical formulas that treat carbuncles, furuncles, and malignant lesions often have viola as one of their main ingredients. Viral infections such as mumps may also be treated with viola.

Herbal Formulas

For long-term use, it is always best to use well-designed herbal formulas, not single herbs. The following are herbal formulas the author has developed with leading authorities. They have been used in thousands of clinics in North America. These formulas contain tonic herbs that are usually used to promote overall health. They are typically used for several months or longer depending upon the advice of your health professional.

Astra 8

Astra 8 is an excellent daily tonic and immune regulator. Astra 8 contains astragalus *(huang qi),* an herb that has been the subject of much research because of its immune-enhancing ability. It was used in the Immune Enhancement Project in San Francisco, California, and in a Transfusion Safety Study at the University of Miami, Florida.

Some of the herbs contained in this formula appear to have a homeostatic effect on the immune system. A deficient immune function may be strengthened or an overactive immune response may be calmed. Astragalus has been shown to have significant anti-viral activity and contains adaptogens, which help alleviate a depressed immune system. All of the herbs in the formula are Qi tonics that support astragalus with the intention of boosting the immune and energy systems. Ganoderma Reishi *(ling zhi)* is included for its immune-enhancing effects. Schizandra *(wu wei zi)* combined with eleuthero root *(ci wu jia)* promote body energy and mental activity while protecting the liver from chronic viral infections. Codonopsis *(dang shen)* and licorice *(gan cao)* together treat immune deficiency and autoimmune disorders. Ligustrum *(nu zhen zi)* promotes circulation and removes toxins from the liver, and also has immune-enhancing properties. Oryza *(gu ya)* aids in digestion.

Astra Isatis

Astra Isatis formula is designed for patients with weak constitutions who are prone to many infections. Astra Isatis was used in a study on immune system enhancement at John Bastyr Naturopathic College in Seattle, Washington. The cooling and warming properties of the herbs are balanced in Astra Isatis to provide long-term therapy for chronic viral infections, which tend to exhaust the Qi and yang.

Astra Isatis combines isatis *(da qing ye* and *ban lan gen),* an herb with strong anti-bacterial and anti-viral properties, with Qi, yin, and yang tonics. The formula contains herbs that help calm an overactive metabolism and inhibit the agitating effects of pathogenic organisms. It includes spleen and kidney tonic herbs chosen for their immune-enhancing properties and their ability to reduce inflammations. Laminaria *(kun bu)* regulates the thyroid and resolves lymphatic congestion. Bupleurum *(chai hu)* invigorates liver qi and is used in the treatment of prolonged infections. Astragalus *(huang qi),* codonopsis *(dang shen),* white atractylodes *(bai zhu),* and dioscorea *(shan yao)* strengthen the spleen, and have immune-enhancing properties according to Western research. Epimedium *(yin yang huo)* tonifies kidney yin and yang. Lycium *(gou qi zi)* nourishes kidney yin. Licorice *(gan cao)* tonifies the adrenal gland and has detoxifying properties.

CordySeng

CordySeng tonifies both yin and yang, strengthens the spleen, stomach, kidneys, and lungs, and helps digestion. CordySeng is especially good for the chronic fatigue found in chronic hepatitis, AIDS, and various types of cancer. It combines the best of the Fu Zheng *(Restore the Normal)* herbs, Qi tonics, and yin tonics. It is designed to be used on its own as an energy tonic and immunomodulating formula or as an adjunct to other herbal formulas. Cordyceps is used in many Chinese cancer-support formulas. It has been shown to increase natural interferon levels in animal cells.

The main ingredient in this formula, Cordyceps *(dong chong xia cao),* is considered a tonic and supporting herb that restores energy, promotes longevity, and improves quality of life. Ganoderma *(reishi; ling zhi)* contains highly active polysaccharides, which appear to have potent immune-regulating effects. It is traditionally used to protect the liver from damage, reduce the symptoms of hepatitis, and lower liver enzyme levels. Astragalus *(huang qi)* and licorice *(gan cao)* have anti-viral and immune-potentiating activity; American ginseng *(xi yang shen)* and ginger *(sheng jiang)* support digestive functions.

Eight Treasures

This formula is indicated for lack of both Qi and blood. The formula is the combination of two smaller formulas, the *Four Gentlemen (si jun zi tang)* to tonify Qi, and the *Four Substances (si wu tang)* to tonify blood. This is one of the most frequently used herbal preparations in traditional Chinese medicine. The formula is particularly indicated for Qi and blood deficiency.

Eight Treasures formula contains codonopsis *(dang shen)* to tonify the Qi while rehmannia *(shu di huang)* nourishes the blood. White atractylodes *(bai zhu)* and poria *(fu ling)* strengthen the spleen and remove dampness thereby assisting codonopsis. White peony *(bai shao)* and tang kuei *(dang gui)* nourish the blood and assist rehmannia in this capacity. An additional herb, spatholobus (millettia, *ji xue teng),* has been added to enhance the formula's ability to both move and tonify the blood. Along with ligusticum *(chuan xiong),* the formula now takes on the increased ability to create new blood, making it valuable to athletic performers, who tend to have exhausted blood. Baked licorice *(zhi gan cao)* tonifies the Qi and harmonizes the middle burner. Ginger *(gan jiang)* and red date *(da zao)* regulate the absorbing function of the spleen and stomach.

Enhance

Enhance is comprised solely of Chinese herbs and is the base formula used in the Quan Yin Herbal Program for HIV-positive persons. It has been designed by Misha Cohen, OMD, L.Ac., based on her experience and the experience at the Quan Yin Healing Arts Center in treating thousands of HIV-positive patients. It was subject to a double-blind clinical study and shown to improve the patients' quality of life. The formula differs from other approaches used in that it is designed to be easier to digest (it protects the spleen and stomach) and contains a greater percentage of herbs that are believed to have anti-bacterial and anti-viral activity according to Chinese and American research. Enhance also has a higher percentage of herbs to tonify and vitalize blood because of the crucial nature of protecting and strengthening the bone marrow in HIV-positive persons.

The main ingredient, Ganoderma *(reishi; ling zhi),* is a Qi tonic that appears to contain one of the most highly active polysaccharides found in mushrooms. Ganoderma has been used in China to treat hepatitis and cancer. Ganoderma and astragalus *(huang qi)* have been shown in Chinese research to be strongly immune enhancing. Other Qi tonics are included for their apparent immune-enhancing and energy-strengthening effects according to research.

A concentrated isatis extract is used in high doses for its strong anti-viral activity, particularly in hepatitis, herpes simplex, herpes zoster, and viral warts. It has a broad range of safety. Additionally, a high proportion of clear heat clean toxin herbs are used for the underlying heat inflammation/viral infection present in persons with HIV infection, cytomegalovirus (CMV), and other chronic viral syndromes.

Spatholobus (millettia, *ji xue teng)* extract was chosen for its clinically shown ability to help increase bone marrow function, thereby assisting in the formation of white blood cells and red blood cells. It is used extensively in China to treat the bone-marrow-suppression effects of chemotherapy. Similarly, it appears to be helpful to people with HIV for treating the side effects of drug therapy such as AZT anemia. Other blood tonics and blood vitalizers in the formula appear to be important in the strengthening of the immunity through stimulating and protecting the bone marrow.

Enhance® contains: Ganoderma (reishi) fruiting body *(ling zhi)*, Isatis extract leaf and root *(ban lan gen* and *da qing ye)*, Spatholobus root/stem *(ji xue teng)*, Astragalus root *(huang qi)*, Tremella fruiting body *(bai mu er)*, Andrographis herb *(chuan xin lian)*, Lonicera flower *(jin yin hua)*, Aquilaria sinensis wood *(chen xiang)*, Epimedium herb *(yin yang huo)*, Oldenlandia herb *(bai hua she she cao)*, Cistanche salsa herb *(rou cong rong)*, Lycium fruit *(gou qi zi)*, Laminaria leaf *(kun bu)*, Tang Kuei root *(dang gui)*, Hu-chang herb *(hu chang)*, American Ginseng root *(xi yang shen)*, Schizandra fruit *(wu wei zi)*, Ligustrum fruit *(nu zhen zi)*, White

Atractylodes rhizome *(bai zhu)*, Rehmannia (cooked) root *(shu di huang)*, Salvia root *(dan shen)*, Curcuma tuber *(yu jin)*, Viola herb/root *(zi hua di ding)*, Citrus peel *(chen pi)*, White Peony root *(bai shao)*, Ho-shou-wu root *(he shou wu)*, Eucommia bark *(du zhong)*, Cardamon fruit *(sha ren)*, Licorice root *(gan cao)*

Marrow Plus®

This formula is based on the clinical experience of Misha Cohen, OMD, L.Ac., in treating persons with AIDS and cancer who are receiving chemotherapeutic agents that suppress bone marrow function. This formula is used in the Quan Yin Herbal Program for HIV-positive persons as an adjunct to Enhance. It will be researched at UCSF, supported by a grant from the NIH Office of Alternative Medicine and Health Concerns.

The chief herb spatholobus (millettia, *ji xue teng*) both vitalizes and tonifies blood. In China this herb is commonly used during cancer therapy to stimulate bone marrow function when it is suppressed by radiation or chemotherapy. *Ho-shou-wu* nourishes the blood and replenishes liver and kidney essence. Salvia *(dan shen)* moves blood and eliminates blood stasis in addition to promoting the repair and regeneration of tissues. Codonopsis *(dang shen)* and astragalus *(huang qi)* replenish Qi and strengthen spleen and stomach function, which is necessary to the production of blood. Both herbs are known to increase white blood cell count. Codonopsis in particular is used in China to treat patients with low WBCs due to radiation or chemotherapy, and is also administered to increase RBCs. The rehmannias *(shu di huang* and *sheng di huang)* nourish essence and strengthen the kidney, so that blood is regenerated. Tang kuei is a strong blood tonic, and helps increase the body's folic acid and vitamin B12 levels, so that anemia is alleviated in many cases. Lycium *(gou qi zi)* nourishes the blood. Lotus seed *(lian zi),* citrus *(chen pi),* red date *(da zao),* and oryza *(gu ya)* strengthen the spleen and aid in the digestion of the formula's herbs. Gelatinum *(E jiao)* strengthens the blood and essence and has been shown to increase RBCs and hemoglobin. This formula may also be used for neuropathy, since salvia *(dan shen)* and other herbs in the formula are known to promote microcirculation.

In order to boost bone marrow function, it is necessary to both vitalize and tonify blood, a specific action required for this type of anemia. Spleen qi and kidney yang should also be tonified.

Six Gentlemen

This is the classic Chinese formula that treats deficiency of spleen qi. Its basis is four herbs (the *Four Gentlemen)* that tonify the Qi of both the spleen and lung. Codonopsis *(dang shen)* and white atractylodes *(bai zhu)* combined tonify the spleen qi and the lung qi, dry dampness, and facilitate the transporting function of the spleen. Poria *(fu ling)* leaches out dampness. Baked licorice *(zhi gan cao)* tonifies the spleen while harmonizing the middle burner (stomach/spleen). Two additional herbs address phlegm: pinellia *(ban xia)* and citrus *(chen pi)* are drying and are able to transform phlegm. Since the formula tends to be cloying, vladimiria souliei *(mu xiang)* and cardamon *(sha ren)* have been added to disperse stagnation in the stomach, facilitating the absorption of the formula.

This formula addresses a wide range of complaints. The key to its proper use lies in identifying deficiency syndromes of the spleen and lung—that is, Qi deficiency. Since the spleen's function in Chinese medicine is to transport dampness, the formula is effective not only as a digestive tonic, but also in treating fatigue, tired limbs, and low energy.

Phlegm is a frequent problem in cases of spleen qi deficiency. Six Gentlemen's function is to dry the spleen and transform phlegm. It is helpful in cases when phlegm turbidity manifests through the lung and its related orifice, the nose. The formula is warming and is thus appropriate for deficient cold type conditions. Yellow or green phlegm indicates heat, a presentation that is NOT appropriate for this formula.

Tremella & American Ginseng

This formula was designed by Misha Cohen, OMD, L.Ac., based on her clinical experience and the experience of the Quan Yin Healing Arts Center in treating thousands of HIV-positive patients.

Tremella & American Ginseng is a formula specifically for individuals with chronic viral syndromes, such as HIV, chronic fatigue immune dysfunction syndrome (CFIDS), and herpes, among others. This formula is used for signs of yin deficiency heat, the symptoms of which may include fatigue, digestive disorders, inability to concentrate, swollen lymph nodes, chronic dry cough, spontaneous sweating, and the like.

The chief herb in the formula is tremella *(bai mu er),* which enriches the yin, moistens the lung, nourishes the stomach, and produces fluids. The deputy herb is American ginseng *(xi yang shen),* which benefits the lung yin, clears deficiency fire, and produces fluids. Individuals who have chronic viral infections generally present a pattern of yin deficiency and exuberant heat because such protracted conditions consume yin and fluids. Thus, these two herbs are aimed at relieving the deficiency heat pattern and at treating dry cough due to lung deficiency and lung heat, a primary symptom in these individuals.

Astragalus *(huang qi)* tonifies the spleen and augments the protective Qi, and stabilizes the exterior; it is used for deficiency with spontaneous sweating. Schizandra *(wu wei zi)* addresses coughing/wheezing due to patterns of lung and kidney deficiency, and inhibits spontaneous sweating and generates fluids. Another major herb in this formula is raw rehmannia *(sheng di huang),* which clears heat and cools the blood, nourishes the yin and generates fluids, and cools the upward-blazing of heart fire. Lycium fruit *(gou qi zi)* is another important herb in that it nourishes and tonifies the liver and kidney yin, since many individuals with chronic viral conditions have yin deficiency of these two organs.

Herbs in this formula that clear heat are lycium bark *(di gu pi),* isatis extract *(ban lan gen* and *da qing ye),* lonicera *(jin yin hua),* and viola *(zi hua di ding)*; the latter three have been found through research to have anti-viral effects as well. Ganoderma *(reishi; ling zhi)* is a general tonifying herb. Herbs that tonify the yin include ophiopogon *(mai men dong),* ephemerantha fimbriata *(shi hu),* ligustrum *(nu zhen zi),* glehnia *(sha shen),* and tortoise shell (from chinemys reevesii) *(gui ban).* Herbs that tonify the yang are cuscuta *(tu si zi)* and epimedium *(yin yang huo)*; those that invigorate the blood are spatholobus (millettia, *ji xue teng),* tang kuei *(dang gui),* and curcuma *(yu jin).* Because of the number of tonifying herbs in the formula, citrus *(chen pi)* and cardamon *(sha ren)* are added to facilitate their digestion and absorption, and licorice *(gan cao)* harmonizes the ingredients.

Immune Nutrients

In addition to eating a diet that contains fresh fruits and vegetables and lean sources of protein, nutritional supplementation can be very important. Numerous studies show that taking a multiple vitamin and mineral supplement enhances immune function in the elderly. Free radical damage—caused by stress, radiation, infection, and chronic illness—depletes the thymus and causes oxidative damage. Antioxidant vitamins and herbs help correct these states. The most important antioxidant nutrients are carotenes, vitamins C and E, zinc, and selenium. These, along with folic acid, B vitamins, and vitamin A, are important for proper immune functioning. Foods that are high in antioxidant activity include berries, broccoli, tomatoes, red grapes, garlic, spinach, tea, carrots, soy, and Neptune krill oil.

Antioxidants

Antioxidants protect the body from "free radicals," molecules that are missing electrons and cause trouble by stealing electrons from other molecules. Antioxidants neutralize the electrical charge to prevent the free radical from taking electrons from other molecules. This process, called oxidation, occurs as a result of normal cell processes, which we can't do much about. For example, it's oxidation at work when metal rusts, or a sliced apple turns brown. But oxidation also occurs as a result of things we can try to minimize, such as stress, UV radiation, alcohol, and exposure to smoke and pollution. Free radicals aren't all bad—they help fight viruses and bacteria, and they help cells communicate with each other—but they are also at work in most chronic disease, particularly cancer, heart disease, and lung disease. Free radicals can damage cell membranes, kill cells directly, or damage DNA so that cells grow out of control, causing cancer.[49]

Antioxidants are found in Neptune krill oil, green tea, lycopene, carotenoids, vitamins C and E, selenium, and zinc, but are in distressingly low supply in the typical modern diet heavy on processed foods. Alpha lipoic acid is one of the premier antioxidants. Because it is both water and fat soluble, it has a wider range of antioxidant activity than vitamins C and E. Alpha lipoic acid also has anti–inflammatory effects, improves oxygen intake, helps regenerate the liver, and helps repair nerve tissue. It is clinically used for the treatment of chemotherapy- and diabetes-induced neuropathy. It helps regulate blood sugar, which is why it is recommended for diabetics. Neptune krill oil, which is available as a supplement, contains naturally occurring antioxidants including astaxanthin. It has more than 300 times the antioxidant capacity of vitamin E.

Vitamins

Vitamin A

Vitamin A has been shown to enhance a number of immune processes including anti-viral and anti-tumor activity, white blood cell function, and antibody response. Vitamin A should not be used in amounts over 5,000 IU by pregnant women; dosages over 25,000 IU per day should only be taken under professional supervision.

A safer option is the use of **carotenes.** Carotenes are the reason that fruits and vegetables have vibrant red, yellow, and orange colors. Mixed carotene supplements containing vitamin A, beta-carotene, alpha-carotene, and lycopene are highly recommended. Carotenes are used for detoxification, aiding the immune system, and improving growth and reproduction. Several carotenoids— including lycopene, beta-carotene, lutein, and canthaxanthin— have been shown to have cancer-preventing properties. In a study at the University of Illinois, lycopene was shown to reduce PSA levels and oxidative cell damage. Additionally, Harvard researchers who evaluated 124,000 patients reported that people who consumed the most lycopene and other carotenoids had a 20–25 percent reduced risk of lung cancer.[50] Carotenoids intake has also been shown to reduce the likelihood of breast cancer. At the

163

New York University School of Medicine, the risk of breast cancer for subjects with low blood levels of carotenoids was twice that of subjects with the highest blood level of carotenoids.[51] Lutein from dietary sources had a protectant effect against colon cancer in a study of 1,993 case subjects with colon cancer and 2,410 control subjects conducted at the University of Utah Medical School.[52]

Folic Acid and B Vitamins

Although it is best known for preventing birth defects, **folic acid** is also important in the immune system. Without folic acid, cells don't divide normally, and so B vitamins and folic acid have important cancer-protective effects. High-dose folic acid (10 mg. per day) normalizes Pap smears in patients with cervical dysplasia, a precancerous condition. In a study conducted by the Albert Einstein College of Medicine in Bronx, New York, based on 295 cancer cases and 5,334 controls, researchers concluded that the women with the highest intakes of folic acid were least likely to develop colorectal cancer.[53] Another study concluded that pregnant women taking folic acid had a reduced risk of giving birth to children with lymphoblastic leukemia.[54] Laboratory experiments have also shown that folic acid and B6 tend to reduce tumor proliferation.

Folic acid deficiency can result from prescription medications and alcohol. Folic acid deficiency may result in poor growth, diarrhea, anemia, and abnormal Pap smears. Patients with candidiasis, Crohn's disease, fatigue, hepatitis, infertility, and ulcerative colitis may have reduced levels of folic acid. Typical dosage is 400–800 mcg. per day. Consult a health professional about the use of higher dosages. Epileptics need to be cautious using folic acid, as it may increase seizures.

Vitamin B$_6$ deficiency results in depressed immune function, whereas B$_{12}$ deficiency interferes with white blood cell function. Thiamine (B$_1$), riboflavin (B$_2$), and pantothenic acid (B$_5$) deficiencies lead to reduced immune response and atrophy of thymus and lymph tissue.[55]

Vitamin C

Numerous clinical studies have shown that vitamin C reduces the frequency, duration, and severity of the common cold. It enhances white blood cell response, fights viral infections, improves thymus functions, and improves mucous membrane linings. The regular use of vitamin C has been shown to lower the risk of certain digestive cancers by 40 percent, according to a study conducted by Yale University. In this study, of 1,095 patients diagnosed with either esophageal or stomach cancer and 687 healthy patients,[56] vitamin C reduced cancer progression.

Sheldon Pinnell, M.D., professor of dermatology at Duke University Medical Center, has found that applied to the skin before UV exposure, vitamin C prevents UV-induced skin damage. This new form of vitamin C, ascorbic palmitate, is fat soluble, and therefore has a longer action than other forms of vitamin C.[57]

Vitamin D

Vitamin D is obtained from sunlight and supplements, and is also found in cod-liver oil. Vitamin D deficiency is common in inflammatory and autoimmune diseases. Vitamin D deficiency has been found in 48 percent of patients with multiple sclerosis,[58] 50 percent of patients with fibromyalgia and lupus,[59] and 62 percent of the morbidly obese[60] (obesity is associated with lowered immune function). It is also common in patients with Graves' disease, ankylosing spondylitis, and rheumatoid arthritis. W. B. Grant, M.D., estimates that 23,000–47,000 cancer deaths might be prevented in the U.S. if sunshine or supplements were used to raise vitamin D levels.[61] Vitamin D helps the body detoxify a bile acid, lithocholic acid, which has been found to cause colon cancer in laboratory experiments. Although not necessarily a therapy for colon cancer, vitamin D, taken in the correct dosage, may have a preventive effect.

The oral dose of vitamin D depends upon sun exposure, body weight, skin pigmentation (dark-skinned people need more sunlight than light-skinned people to raise vitamin D levels), diet, medication usage, and digestive absorption. Up to 4,000 IU per day may be indicated for optimal immune function—however, we suggest having a health professional monitor your vitamin D levels, for dosages above 800 IU per day.[62]

Vitamin E

Studies show that supplemental vitamin E can reduce risk for cancer and enhance immune functions. According to research conducted by the National Cancer Institute, vitamin E, in the form of alpha-Tocopherol, reduces the risk for prostate cancer. It has been hypothesized that alpha-Tocopherol suppresses PSA (prostate-specific antigen), a marker for tumor growth. According to research conducted in Poland, reviewing 180 cases of colorectal cancer and 80 cases of gastric cancer, there was an inverse correlation between vitamin E intake and gastric cancer.[63]

Supplemental vitamin E has been found to increase CD-4 (T-helper) cells, an important indicator of immune function. Eight patients over age sixty-five were given vitamin E for 235 days at doses of 60 IU, 200 IU, and 800 IU, and showed T-helper cell increases of 25, 58, and 65 percent, respectively. There were no adverse reports noted.[64]

Natural vitamin E in the form of d-alpha tocopherol or mixed natural tocopherols is recommended over the synthetic form called dl-alpha tocopherol, which is cheaper and less active. Foods that contain natural vitamin E include wheat germ oil, nuts, seeds, vegetable oil, egg yolks, and leafy green vegetables.

Colostrum

Colostrum is the clear fluid that precedes milk in the hours after a mammal gives birth. This nutrient is rich in protein and anti-bacterial constituents, as well as immunoglobulins. Colostrum is useful for stopping diarrhea, and may have anti-inflammatory properties. Colostrum is typically used for intestinal disease, slow-healing wounds, and people who are frequently sick. It is also used for skin disease, particularly when applied topically. Bovine colostrum preparations are pasteurized or micro-filtered to prevent the risk of contamination. Dosage is 2,000–3,000 mg. per day in divided doses. This dosage is usually reduced after two weeks, or if the patient develops constipation. Colostrum is well tolerated by most people who have dairy sensitivity, and can be used, over time, to heal the intestines and make them less sensitive.

Co Q-10 (Coenzyme Q-10)

Although best know as a treatment for cardiovascular conditions, Co Q-10 is necessary for optimal function of the immune system. In a clinical protocol, thirty-two patients with high-risk breast cancer were treated with antioxidants, essential fatty acids, and 90 mg. of Co Q-10. Six of the thirty-two patients showed tumor regression. In one case, the dosage of Co Q-10 was increased to 390 mg. After one month, a mammogram confirmed the absence of the tumor. Another patient who received the high-dose Co Q-10 got similar results.[65] Although two cases do not mean that Co Q-10 reduces tumors, Co Q-10 does support toxin removal, and cancer causes toxins to accumulate. It is also recommended for anyone on the chemotherapy drug Adriamycin. Adriamycin depletes Co Q-10 levels in the heart, which can lead to heart damage. Look for highly absorbable forms of Co Q-10, or use it with fish oil to improve absorption.

Enzymes

Enzymes are traditionally used at mealtimes to improve digestive function. Today, enzymes may also be used for a wide variety of inflammatory and digestive ailments, including pancreatic insufficiency disease, celiac disease, lactose intolerance, food allergies, sinusitis, pancreatitis, injuries, lymphedema, MS, and experimentally in cancer. Enzymes have been found in animal tests to improve nutrient absorption and prevent weight loss, which can be a considerable concern in immune disorders.[66] Enzymes are also useful in treating inflammatory conditions, such as rheumatoid arthritis, by restoring normal blood flow, reducing swelling, and accelerating the healing response.[67]

Enzymes can be derived from plant sources, such as bromelain from pineapple, or from animal sources, such as pancreatic enzymes. A combination of bromelain, pancreatin, trypsin, and chymotrypsin are particularly good for treating inflammatory disorders, and should be taken on an empty stomach. Papaya enzymes are used to assist digestion. Enzymes from fungus, wheat, and rice are usually taken with meals. Follow the label directions for dosage.

Fish Oil/EPA and DHA

More than two thousand studies have been published in medical journals on the health benefits of omega-3 fatty acids found in fish oils. These studies show that fish oil reduces several inflammatory markers, protects the heart, and may reduce asthma and arthritis symptoms and cancer risk. According to University of California cell biologist Bruce Ames, Ph.D., 30 percent of cancers result from chronic inflammation and chronic infections.[68]

Paul Terry, Ph.D., and his colleagues at the Karolinska Institute in Sweden measured the health of 6,000 male twins. They found that men who regularly ate fish had up to half the risk of prostate cancer compared to those who ate no fish.[69] According to an Australian study, as little as one meal including fish per week significantly reduced the likelihood of asthma. In a study of 63 patients with rheumatoid arthritis, men and women taking fish oil capsules containing 1.7 g. of EPA and 1 g. DHA experienced reduced pain and were able to reduce their use of pain-relieving medication. Fish rich diets also protect the heart. In an 800-patient study at the University of Washington, one fish meal weekly reduced the risk of cardiac arrest by half.[70]

Neptune krill oil is my favorite form of fish oil. Krill oil offers EPA and DHA that's more bioavailable, or usable by your body, than most fish oils. Instead of taking 10 capsules a day to get a therapeutic dose, as is necessary with most fish oils, you need to take only 3 capsules a day. Plus, krill oil doesn't cause the digestive side effects, such as regurgitation, bloating, and bad breath, commonly experienced with fish oils. Cod-liver oil in liquid form is not likely to cause digestive problems either, and is also a rich source of vitamin D. Although I am unaware of any vegetarian sources of EPA, DHA supplements derived from algae are available; however, they do not have the wide range of benefits associated with fish oil preparations containing EPA/DHA.

Because fish oil thins the blood, it makes sense to be monitored by your health professional if you are taking prescription blood thinners such as Coumadin.

Grape Seed Extract/Plant Flavonoids

Grape seed extract contains antioxidant compounds called oligomeric proanthocyanidins (OPCs), which are also found in pine bark, lemon tree bark, cranberries, and citrus peels. Proanthocyanidins have a wide range of activity. They are important to connective tissue, have anti-inflammatory effects through antioxidant activity, and prevent the release of inflammatory compounds such as histamines, prostaglandins, and leukotrienes. At Creighton University, grape seed extract was found to have greater antioxidant protection than vitamin C, vitamin E, and beta-carotene. The extract was found to have a cancer-killing effect toward human breast, lung, and gastric cancer cells while improving normal cells.[71]

NAC

NAC, or N-acetylcysteine, is a form of the amino acid cysteine, which enhances production of the enzyme glutathione. Glutathione levels are often low in people with immune conditions. Some researchers theorize that NAC's antioxidant effects may be helpful in preventing cataracts and macular degeneration, lowering cancer risk, and slowing the progression of MS and Parkinson's disease. Conventional physicians commonly use NAC to break up mucus in people with respiratory ailments. Studies have shown that NAC inhibits reproduction of some viruses, and that HIV-positive patients taking NAC were twice as likely to survive for two years as those not taking NAC. NAC has also been shown to reduce levels of substances associated with heart disease.[72]

Probiotics

Probiotics are good bacteria that live in the gastrointestinal tract, and are thought to inhibit the growth of harmful bacteria basically by crowding them out. Probiotics are especially important during and after the use of antibiotics. Antibiotics wipe out both the good and the bad bacteria, making the body susceptible to diarrhea, fungal overgrowth, and urinary tract infections. Other uses of probiotics include preventing traveler's diarrhea, reducing indigestion and intestinal gas, and treating gastrointestinal side effects of chemo and radiation therapy.

Lactobacillus acidophilus and Bifidobacterium bifidum are the best known probiotics. Probiotics can be either taken as food, in the form of homemade yogurt and miso. Probiotics should be taken on an empty stomach, preferably before bed. If you are taking antibiotics or other medication, take probiotics at least two hours before or after your medications. In our clinic, we have found three brands particularly good: PB8, Natren, and Culturelle.

Quercetin

Quercetin is a bioflavonoid found in citrus fruits, apples, red grapes, and green vegetables, and is best known for the anti-allergic effects it achieves by suppressing histamine release. Quercetin is also currently being studied for its cancer-inhibiting effects. In a study published in the *Journal of Hyperthermia,* quercetin, in conjunction with high heat therapy, or hyperthermia, inhibited cancer growth and amplified the effects of hyperthermia on two types of prostate cancer. Quercetin has been found to increase the efficacy of the chemotherapy drug cisplain. Also, taking quercetin with Adriamycin reduces the dosage needed, important because Adriamycin is highly toxic and can cause heart problems.[73]

Selenium

Selenium is essential for the proper functioning of the immune system, and may protect against cancer. Selenium supplements stimulate white blood cell and thymus function, and also enhance interleukin-2, a naturally occurring immune-building compound. All diseases of aging are influenced by selenium, and it may protect against cancer. Selenium works closely with vitamin E in the production of antibodies, the binding of toxic metals, and the promotion of normal growth and fertility. Selenium ensures adequate oxygen supply in the heart. Low levels of selenium are related to leukemia, bladder, colon, ovarian, prostate, lung, and prostate cancer.

Selenium activates an antioxidant enzyme called glutathione peroxidase, which may have a role in cancer protection. In one clinical trial, patients who took 200 mcg. selenium supplements daily showed a 50 percent lower incidence of lung, colon, and prostate cancer than patients not taking selenium supplements.[74] Additional studies have shown selenium can help people with oral, ovarian, bowel, and skin cancer.[75] Selenium also has a protective effect against chemotherapy, kidney toxicity, and bone marrow suppression.[76] Thirty-one patients with ovarian cancer undergoing the chemotherapy regimen of cisplatin and cyclophosphamide received a supplement that contained a daily dosage of

60 mg. of beta–carotene, 800 mg. of vitamin C, 144 mg. of vit-amin E, 18 mg. of riboflavin, and 190 mg. of niacin. Half the patients were randomly assigned to the selenium group. The selenium group received 200 mcg. per day. After three months, white blood cell count was significantly higher in the selenium group than in the nonselenium group. After three months of supplementation, nausea, hair loss, intestinal gas, abdominal pain, weakness, malaise, vomiting, stomatitis, and loss of appetite were each significantly lower in the patients who received selenium.

Researchers are also looking at selenium in relation to supporting the immune system in HIV-positive people. A study of almost 1,000 HIV-positive Tanzanian women concluded that low plasma selenium levels were associated with a higher risk of mortality.[77]

Food sources of selenium include brewer's yeast, organ and muscle meats, fish, Brazil nuts, broccoli, cabbage, cucumbers, radishes, garlic, and onions. Typical supplement dosage is 200–400 mcg. per day.

Zinc

Zinc promotes the destruction of foreign microorganisms, boosts CD-4 (T cell) counts, reduces harmful free radicals, and activates the thymus, the major gland in our immune system. Zinc also inhibits several viruses including the common cold and herpes simplex virus. Typical dosage is 15–60 mg. daily. Amounts over 100 mg. may be contraindicated, especially for long-term usage.

Chapter Three

Conditions and Treatments

In this chapter I discuss various immune conditions that can be treated with different natural methods. Many of the products mentioned under Self-Help can be found in health food stores or pharmacies. Products listed under Professional Treatment are available through health professionals, as they are more potent and treat specific syndrome patterns. In undertaking any treatment it is important to be patient in giving these natural remedies time to exert their effects. One should also be mindful that what works for one person may not work for another with the same biomedical condition. This is why health professionals experienced with these remedies and therapies can provide invaluable guidance. Whenever possible, natural therapies should be undertaken under the guidance of a health professional. Typically your herbalist selects the most appropriate herbs and formulas based upon your symptoms, constitution, tongue and pulse.

In general, herbs and supplements work best for chronic conditions. For acute immune conditions, biomedical solutions such as antibiotics work more quickly and more effectively than natural methods.

Included under various conditions are case histories to illustrate the benefits of natural remedies in treating these diseases. In most cases natural approaches can be combined with standard methods.

Addison's Disease (Primary Adrenal Insufficiency)

Addison's disease occurs when the adrenal glands don't produce enough cortisol, and in some cases, aldosterone. Most cases of Addison's disease are autoimmune in nature, a result of the immune system making antibodies that attack the adrenal glands and slowly destroy them. Cortisol helps the body respond to stress, and the amount of cortisol produced in the body is precisely balanced. The symptoms of Addison's disease come on slowly, and include chronic, worsening fatigue and muscle weakness, weight loss, low blood pressure, nausea, vomiting, and a characteristic darkening of the skin that looks like a suntan, but affects unexposed parts of the body, and is most apparent on scars, on the lips, at joints, and on mucous membranes. Addison's disease is treated by replacing the missing cortisol with hydrocortisone tablets taken once or twice a day, and if aldosterone is deficient, with oral fludrocortisone acetate.[1]

Self-Help

◆ B vitamins including pantothenic acid (use as directed)

Professional Treatment

- Adrenosen (2 tablets three times per day) helps to rebuild the adrenal gland
- Astra 8 (3 tablets three times per day) contains herbs to help the body adapt to stress
- Chzyme (2 tablets three times per day) for indigestion
- Licorice 25, a high-dose licorice preparation, may help reduce the need for hydrocortisone tablets (1 tablet three times per day)

Allergies and Hay Fever

One out of three people in the U.S. has allergies. Allergies often run in families and are growing in prevalence. One of the theories about the rise in allergies is the hygiene hypothesis, which suggests that by reducing our exposure to bacteria, our bodies may overreact to harmless substances such as pollen. Additional possibilities include the use of antacids, which suppress immune function, the reduction in breast-feeding, less physical activity, pollutants, items found in new homes (including carpeting and particle board furniture), and first- and secondhand cigarette smoke. Normally, the immune system defends the body against foreign substances. However, for people who are susceptible to allergens, the body reacts physically with common allergic reactions including runny nose, sneezing, watery eyes, skin rash, and itchy eyes and skin. Swelling may also occur. Asthma may be triggered by allergies. Seasonal allergies, commonly known as hay fever, result from airborne particles such as pollens that occur only during part of the year.

Particularly sensitive individuals can react more dramatically with anaphylactic reactions that require immediate medical attention, with symptoms including difficulty breathing and falling blood pressure. Blood tests can be performed to measure eosinophils, a type of white blood cell that is produced in large numbers during an allergic reaction, along with other tests to identify allergens that provoke a reaction.

The primary treatment for allergies is to avoid the allergen, whether it's a particular food, animal, chemical, or drug. In the past, sensitive patients were advised to move to climates where there were fewer plants likely to cause allergic reactions, such as the Southwest, but this option is no longer viable because of the introduction of nonnative, symptom-producing plants in these areas. Installing air filters can help, particularly in the bedroom. Allergy shots may be administered; however, these are not always effective and often this regimen may take more than three years to complete. Physicians more typically prescribe medication such as antihistamines or steroids. An over-the-counter medicine, Chromolyn, is an effective nasal spray that inhibits mast cells, thus reducing or eliminating allergic reactions. It is also available by prescription. If you suffer from a serious allergic reaction, it is best to carry a syringe of epinephrine (adrenaline), as well as antihistamine tablets.

There are many complementary approaches to treating allergies. For example, professionally administered herbs can be prescribed as a long-term approach to reduce allergic symptoms. This can be very effective for seasonal allergies, and may be worth trying for food and skin allergies. Other approaches may include homeopathy, nutritional medicine, and body-mind treatments such as NAET *(Nambudripad's Allergy Elimination Techniques)*. The rotation diet (see Chapter Four, "Digestive Clearing Diet") may also be appropriate for reducing allergic symptoms related to foods. Avoiding histamine-containing foods and beverages including alcoholic beverages, fish, and aged food will help many people with seasonal allergies. Nose guards and portable air filters are also good, especially if air conditioning is not available.

According to Chinese medicine theory, some allergic conditions—such as allergic rhinitis or hay fever—are classified as wind syndromes because they erupt and subside rapidly. Wind-relieving herbs such as xanthium *(cang er zi)*, ephedra *(ma huang)*, and cinnamon twig *(gui zhi)* elevate serum IgG to neutralize allergens, and increase the T cell ratio. Other herbs, such as scute *(huang qin)*, inhibit the release of histamines. Scute also works to inhibit delayed hypersensitivity by enhancing the phagocytic action of white blood cells to absorb allergens. Other herbs such as forsythia *(lian qiao)* and perilla *(zi su ye)* work to eliminate antigens.

Sophora *(ku shen)* is traditionally used to treat eczema and allergic dermatitis. Laboratory research has shown that it increases the intracellular content of cAMP, an important substance that mediates hormonal effects, by inhibiting phosphodiesterase, and thus preventing mast cells from releasing the chemicals that cause allergic reactions.

Blood-activating herbs such as tang kuei *(dang gui)*, salvia *(dan shen)*, and motherwort *(yi mu cao)* inhibit IgM and IgG antibodies, and so can be used to treat transfusion reactions, autoimmune or drug-induced hemolytic anemia, and idiopathic thrombocytopenic purpurea (ITP).

Chinese research shows that many herbs are immunomodulators and are considered by some researchers to be adaptogenic, meaning that they help the body regulate itself. For example, Chinese red dates *(da zao)* contain substances that augment ephedra's anti-asthmatic effects. Many tonic herbs improve the quality and quantity of T-helper and T-suppressor cells, thus modulating immune reactions. The traditional formula *Sheng Mai San*—which contains ginseng, ophiopogon, and schizandra—can inhibit delayed hypersensitive reactions and counteracts the immune system suppression caused by chemotherapy.

Self-Help

- Nettles (use as directed)
- Quercetin and other antioxidants (use as directed)
- Butterbur (use as directed)
- NAC (N–acetylcysteine) (500 to 1,000 mg. per day)

Professional Treatment

- Xanthium Relieve Surface (2 tablets three to four times per day) plus Astra C (1 tablet three times per day); this combination works quickly to reduce symptoms. Astra C is typically used long term to build up defensive energy (wei qi)
- Nasal Tabs 2 (3 tablets three to four times per day) used for sinus congestion. For sinus infection with congestion, combine Nasal Tabs 2 with Coptis Purge Fire (2 tablets three to four times per day)
- Six Gentlemen plus Astra 8 used as a long-term tonic
- Clear Phlegm (2 tablets three to four times per day) usually combined with one of the above formulas with copious mucus

Case Study

Joyce was a forty-two-year-old flight attendant who had a life-time of seasonal allergies. In the past year she had contracted two sinus infections and frequently felt like she was coming down with a cold. She reported constant clear, white, and yellow mucus. She used antihistamines every day. She also suffered from cluster headaches. Her pulse was slippery and her tongue was normal with a thick yellow and white coat.

We recommended that she eliminate all dairy products from her diet and that she reduce sweets. We also suggested Clear Phlegm (2 tablets four times per day) and Xanthium Relieve Surface (3 tablets four times per day).

After two weeks she reported that when she followed the diet there was markedly less phlegm. Although she was not aware of it, I also remarked that she did not come into the consultation room with tissues in her hand as she had for her first appointment. Her pulse was less slippery and her tongue less coated.

After one month she started to have a dry throat, so we switched Clear Phlegm to the more tonifying Astra C (2 tablets three times per day). She maintained on Xanthium Relieve Surface and Astra C for three months. She was able to reduce her antihistamine use, and said her headaches were less frequent and less severe.

Amyotrophic Lateral Sclerosis (ALS)

ALS is commonly known in the U.S. as Lou Gehrig's disease, after the New York Yankee baseball player who died from ALS in 1941. It is a disease in which motor nerves die, causing paralysis. Symptoms include tripping and stumbling, loss of muscle control and strength in hands and arms, difficulty speaking, swallowing, or breathing, chronic fatigue, and muscle twitching and cramping. ALS is more common in men, with the average age of onset at fifty-five. Symptoms get progressively worse, and death generally comes from respiratory complications. ALS is almost always fatal, though people with ALS can live for many years, particularly with a ventilator. For example, British physicist

Stephen Hawking has been living with ALS for more than thirty-five years.

Because it's so similar to other neuromuscular diseases, diagnosis of ALS is by process of elimination, and thus time-consuming. MRI (magnetic resonance imaging), EMG (electromyogram), muscle biopsies, and blood tests may be used. A diagnosis of ALS requires damage on both upper and lower motor neurons, with three limbs affected. The FDA-approved drug called Riluzole can slow its progression, while other drugs are prescribed to relieve symptoms.[2] Experimental approaches to halt the progression of ALS include high-dose antioxidant therapy, which may include intravenous nutrients including glutathione, a gluten-free diet, treating ALS with antibiotic regimens as if it were Lyme disease, and supervised detoxification treatments as if the person suffered from toxic exposure.

Professional Treatment

- High-dose antioxidants including glutathione administered intravenously
- Vinpurazine to improve cognitive functioning (2 tablets two times per day)
- Creatine has been shown to be effective in preventing ALS in mice (2 to 10 grams per day)
- Power Mushrooms to maintain immune functioning (3 tablets three times per day)
- EPAQ krill oil (3 soft gel capsules per day with meals)

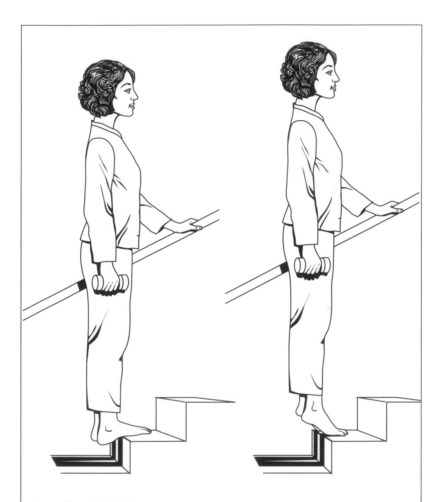

Standing Calf Raise

Stand on the bottom step of a staircase with your feet shoulder width apart, and your heels hanging a few inches over the edge of the step. Hold a weight in one hand, allowing that arm to hang at your side, and support yourself by holding the railing with your other hand. Slowly rise up onto the balls of your feet, lifting your heels as high as possible. Pause. Slowly lower your heels back down to the starting position. As this exercise involves only one weight you might consider using a 5–10 pound weight to start. Do 12–15 repetitions per set, complete three sets.

183

Anemia

There are three types of anemia: iron deficiency anemia, pernicious anemia (a vitamin B_{12} deficiency), and folic acid deficiency.

Iron deficiency anemia often has no symptoms in the initial stages. Left untreated, it may cause fatigue and a pale complexion. Foods that are rich in absorbable iron include meats (especially liver), poultry, fish, eggs, and peas. Supplements may be necessary for women who lose blood during menstruation, vegetarians, or those who do not get enough iron in their diet. A wide range of iron formulas are available in health food stores and pharmacies. At our clinic, we usually recommend liquid iron products because they seem the easiest for most people to digest. *Do not* take iron supplements if you have adequate levels of iron, because excess iron is correlated with heart disease and other serious conditions.

Pernicious anemia, or B_{12} deficiency, is characterized by fatigue, painful tongue, poor appetite, numbness in the hands and feet, memory loss, depression, and dementia. Vitamin B_{12} is common in dairy products and meat, so vegetarians might want to take supplemental B_{12}, or have annual blood tests to test for anemia and B_{12} levels. B_{12} deficiency is best treated by injection. Sublingual (under the tongue) tablets may be the next best option if you can't get B_{12} injections from your physician or HMO, or as a preventive measure.

Folic acid deficiency interferes with the production of red blood cells. There may be fatigue, weight loss, and diarrhea. Folic acid deficiency is most common among alcoholics, pregnant women, and children during growth spurts. Alcohol, medications, liver disease, thyroid imbalance, and smoking all deplete folic acid. Raw fruits and vegetables, liver, and kidney contain folic acid. Folic acid also may be taken in supplement form (800 mcg. per day), or in folic acid–rich foods such as molasses, raisins, and red dates.

Self-Help

◆ Liquid iron (use as directed)
◆ B12 (1,000 mcg. per day or as directed by a health practitioner)
◆ Folic acid (800 mcg. per day or as directed by a health practitioner)

Professional Treatment

◆ Marrow Plus (3 tablets three to four times per day) is used as an adjunct to natural treatments. It builds blood in TCM

Ankylosing Spondylitis

Ankylosing spondylitis is a type of progressive chronic arthritis in which the body makes antibodies that act on the joints in the spine, causing pain and stiffness in the back, neck, and hips.

Ankylosing spondylitis most commonly occurs in men, beginning in adolescence after an infection. Pain is often worse in the morning, and better with activity. Over time, the inflammation may cause the spine to fuse together. The inflammation may affect other joints, the eyes, lungs, and heart valves. Treatment consists of exercise and physical therapy to reduce stiffness, and non-steroidal anti-inflammatory drugs (NSAIDs) such as ibuprofen (Advil, Nuprin, Motrin), naproxen (Aleve), or the newer COX-2 inhibitors (Celebrex) for pain and inflammation.

Professional Treatment

- High-potency antioxidant such as Quercenol and vitamins may help reduce symptoms (use as directed)
- Collagenex helps build up joint integrity and reduces inflammation (2 tablets two times per day)
- Mobility 2 for inflammation and stiffness (3 tablets three times per day)

Anthrax

Anthrax is caused by the *Bacillus anthracis* bacteria. It is highly contagious, and traditionally spread to people from animals, though it has recently been spread through terrorist activities. Although infection is usually introduced through the skin, it can also be acquired by eating contaminated meat or by inhaling spores or bacteria.

Anthrax infection first appears as a skin infection that begins as a reddish brown bump that grows in size, with considerable swelling. The bump blisters and hardens and then the center breaks open. A clear fluid oozes out and a black scab forms. Lymph nodes in the affected area may swell, and the person may have flu symptoms such as fever, muscle aches, headache, nausea, and vomiting.

Inhaled anthrax (pulmonary anthrax) causes the lymph nodes near the lung to break down. Infected fluid builds up in the lungs. At first, the symptoms are similar to the flu, but severe breathing difficulties develop in a few days, followed by shock and coma. Infection of the brain and meningoencephalitis may occur.[3] This form of anthrax is often fatal.

Intestinal anthrax can be fatal if it reaches the bloodstream. The bacteria grow in the wall of the intestine and release a toxin

186

that causes bleeding and tissue death. **Because of the severity of anthrax it is important to seek medical attention immediately.**

Western doctors recommend Cipro, penicillin, and other antibiotics, such as erythromycin. Steroids may be used to reduce lung inflammation. Anthrax vaccine is used by the military and high-risk groups such as postal workers. At the time of writing, the vaccine is not available to the general public because antibiotics are effective, and as with any vaccine, side effects and allergic reactions have been reported. On the basis of animal testing, the vaccine is administered in three dosages over a month's time.

Professional Treatment

- Clear Heat in conjunction with biomedical treatment with heat signs (2 to 3 tablets three times per day)
- Prevent infection with Cordyceps and CordySeng. Cordyceps increases NK cells and helps the body manufacture immune factors. CordySeng contains additional supportive herbs (2 to 3 tablets three times per day)

Asthma

Asthma is characterized by wheezing, shortness of breath, tightness in the chest, and coughing. Respiratory infections, exercise, stress, cold, exposure to allergens, and some medications may aggravate asthma. People with asthma may also be sensitive to sulfites, artificial flavors and colors. Asthma attacks may be mild or life-threatening, which is why it is important to be under the care of a health professional. Physicians diagnose asthma on the basis of a physical exam, breathing and allergy tests, and X-rays.

A peak flow meter can help you monitor your lung function and can help you prevent a flare-up. It should be used several times per day if you are on medication for asthma. Asthma medications include anti-inflammatory drugs such as inhaled steroids, cromolyn, and nedocromil sodium. Beta agonists such as albuterol (Proventil, Ventolin) are inhalants used for acute attacks, and before exercise and exposure to cold air. Salmeterol (Serevent) is a long-acting beta agonist that can prevent airway constriction for up to twelve hours. Theophylline and oral steroids may be prescribed if the above solutions are not satisfactory.

Chinese herbal medicine can be especially helpful for long-term asthma sufferers. By listening to your symptoms, and monitoring your tongue and pulse, your herbalist can recommend tonic herbs that over time may strengthen your immune system, and decrease flare-ups. An acupuncturist can show you points you can press during an acute asthma attack.

Self-Help

- Ginkgo has anti-inflammatory effects (use as directed)
- Magnesium (200 to 600 mg. per day)
- NAC (N-acetylcysteine) (500 to 1,000 mg. per day)

Professional Treatment

- Ginseng and Gecko (3 to 5 tablets three times per day), traditional formula used for chronic asthma due to kidney deficiency
- Xanthium Relieve Surface (3 tablets three times per day) reduces allergic response

- Flavonex (2 to 3 tablets three times per day) contains ginkgo and other anti-inflammatory herbs

Case Studies

Case #1

Judith was a forty-nine-year-old office worker with asthma that was worsening. Her main symptoms were fatigue, wheezing, rattling cough, dry cough, and runny nose in the morning. All symptoms were worse in cold weather. She had been taking Singular and Claritin and using an Albuterol inhaler (two times per day) for several years. Her pulse was rapid, slippery, and deep; her tongue purplish red, with a moist coating. We recommended Ginseng and Gecko (3 tablets three times per day) with Power Mushrooms (2 tablets three times per day). Ginseng and Gecko was selected to help the kidney grasp the Qi and reduce phlegm; Power Mushrooms was selected to tonify Qi, reduce dampness, and strongly improve immune function. After two weeks Judith had less fatigue and slightly less coughing. Her pulse and tongue were unchanged. After being on the protocol for three months Judith's fatigue had disappeared, and all other symptoms were improved. After consulting her doctor she was able to reduce her use of the inhaler. Her pulse was deep, and her tongue looked normal. As she was still having some wheezing and dry cough we switched her protocol to Lily Bulb (3 tablets three times per day) and she remained on Power Mushrooms (2 tablets three times per day). Judith remains on the protocol at the time of this writing.

Case #2

Lauren was a thirty-eight-year-old sales professional. The reason for her visit was that although her asthma was controlled by medications, the cost of these medications was $300 to $400 per month. She was also concerned about side effects. She maintained on steroidal and non-steroidal inhalers, prednisone, theophylline tablets, and an antihistamine. Her main symptoms were coughing and wheezing worsened by exercise or cold air, which were worse in the morning, frequent colds and flu, and hay fever. She characterized her cough as being dry, Lauren's tongue was red with a thin dark-yellow coat, and her pulse was thin and rapid. We recommended NAC (500 mg. three times per day), Tremella & American Ginseng (3 tablets four times per day), and CordySeng (2 tablets four times per day). NAC is used to improve breathing capacity and has strong antioxidant effects, Tremella & American Ginseng is used to clear heat and nourish the lungs, and CordySeng improves breathing capacity and tonifies the lungs.

After two weeks she reported greater physical energy, she was able to breathe deeply without coughing, and she was able to run a few times for the first time in six months. She talked to her doctor, who said it was okay to reduce her use of inhalers, but she should keep them with her in case she had increased coughing or difficulty breathing. Her pulse and tongue were unchanged. She continued on the herbs for the next year, gradually being able to eliminate all her medications, with the exception of her steroid inhaler. As the use of medication decreased, her symptom pattern showed less heat and more deficiency, characterized by a slower pulse and a pale tongue. Therefore, Ginseng and Gecko, which tonifies kidney yang, was substituted for Tremella & American Ginseng.

Bronchitis

Bronchitis is an inflammation of the bronchi usually caused by a virus or bacterial infection. Irritative bronchitis is caused by dust, air pollution, tobacco, and chemicals. Bronchitis starts out like a cold, with the onset of coughing usually signaling the beginning of bronchitis. The cough may start out dry, and shortly after turn up some yellow or green phlegm. In severe cases, a high fever may last three to five days. The cough, wheezing, and shortness of breath, however, may last several weeks. Bronchitis is usually diagnosed on the basis of symptoms. If symptoms persist, or are severe, an X-ray may be needed to rule out pneumonia. Biomedical treatment usually involves resting, drinking plenty of liquids, and taking acetaminophen (Tylenol) or ibuprofen, because aspirin is contraindicated for children. Antibiotics should be used only after a laboratory culture reveals the presence of bacteria.

Self-Help

- Slippery elm can be used to moisten lungs and reduce coughing (1 tsp. one to three times per day in hot water)
- Eucalyptus essential oil or products containing eucalyptus can be applied topically to help reduce chest congestion

Professional Treatment

- Isatis Gold (3 tablets four times per day) to reduce heat and mucus
- Clear Air (3 tablets two to three times per day) stops coughing
- Tremella & American Ginseng (3 to 5 tablets four times per day) used for dry cough
- Clear Phlegm (3 tablets three times per day) reduces phlegm

Case Study

Sandy, a forty-six-year-old therapist, contracted pneumonia in the past six months. More recently she developed bronchitis in the past three months. When we saw her she was battling bronchitis. She had a fever and frequent coughing and also complained of sinus pain and fatigue. She had just finished a second course of antibiotics. Her phlegm was clear. Her pulse was slippery and her tongue was red with a thin yellow coat. We recommended Isatis Gold (3 tablets four times per day) with PB8 acidophilus (2 capsules twice a day). After three days the fever was eliminated, and sinus pain was improved. She complained of a constant low-level coughing, greater fatigue, and phlegm. Sandy's pulse was slow and less slippery, and her tongue was pale and the coating was reduced. We recommended CordySeng at a high dosage (3 tablets three times per day) as well as continuing with acidophilus. CordySeng reduces coughing and strengthens the lungs. After two days Sandy called to say she was all better. We counseled her to continue taking the CordySeng at a high dosage until her next appointment. One week later she looked much better, the coughing was eliminated, and she was no longer tired. Her pulse was normal and her tongue was slightly pale. We suggested she continue taking CordySeng at 3 tablets twice per day. After four months she had not had any lung problems.

Cancer

According to the American Cancer Society, cancer is the second leading cause of death in the U.S. In 2001 there were more than 500,000 cancer deaths, and more than two million newly diagnosed cancer patients. The most common cancers are skin, lung, colorectal, breast, and prostate cancer. The overall five-year survival rate is approximately 59 percent.

The immune system is largely responsible for keeping cancer cells in check—for example, cancer is one hundred times more likely to occur in people taking immune-suppressing drugs.[4] We all carry malignant potential in normal genes known as proto-oncogenes (onco is Greek for tumor). With a weakened immune system or exposure to carcinogenic chemicals, oncogenes may be activated and turn normal cells into cancer cells. If tumor-suppressing genes are absent or not functioning properly, the cancer produced by an undetected oncogene may not be completely suppressed and a tumor may develop. While it's not clear why the immune system doesn't always recognize and attack cancer cells, it has been suggested that oncogenes produce proteins in larger amounts than normal, causing the cells to mutate and send inappropriate messages that confuse the immune system.

Early detection is one of the chief advances in cancer treatment made by biomedical science. For example, the use of lab tests like the Pap test for cervical cancer and PSA (prostate-specific antigen) testing for prostate cancer have greatly decreased mortality from these cancers. Other detection methods, such as examining the skin, can be conducted by both the patient and practitioner. Your doctor can order tests for microscopic traces of blood in the stool and biopsies.

Cancer is difficult to treat because, unlike normal cells, cancer cells can't stop growing. Untreated, they grow out of control, displacing normal cells and competing with them for nutrients. Unchecked, cancer cells may develop into a mass called a tumor, or metastasize, spreading through the blood or lymph system to other areas in the body. Western medicine treats cancer with chemotherapy drugs and radiation, which are toxic, though more toxic to cancer cells than to normal cells. But the effectiveness of these harsh therapies is uncertain and unpredictable, while they also deplete a patient's system, often making them feel far sicker than the cancer does. In addition to killing cancer cells, chemotherapy and radiation treatments can damage healthy tissue, causing nausea, fatigue, and mouth sores. Radiation may burn skin in the area being treated, making it red and irritated, like a sunburn. Chinese and Western herbs can help alleviate some of these side effects. Chinese herbs can also be used to offset damage caused by immune therapies such as interferon or corticosteroid usage.

In the future, we can expect to see the development of cancer treatments that focus on using natural substances, such as human genes and plants, to correct the immune system, and more precise pharmaceutical bullets that target cancer cells while sparing healthy cells. Research has shown that Chinese herbs may offer anti-cancer activity with far fewer side effects than standard chemotherapy treatment. Some herbs kill tumors directly, while others boost the body's immune response, and thus its ability to fight cancer cells itself. Studies have shown that *Sheng Mai San*— a popular Chinese herbal formula whose name means "Generate the Pulse Powder"—stimulates immune functions and inhibits cancer cell growth in the test tube and in animal and human models, and that it also ameliorates the clinical side effects of cancer drugs. Other Chinese herbs have failed to show results in the test tube, but demonstrate significant anti-cancer activity in animal and human models.[5]

According to the American Cancer Society, if you have any of these signs, you should consult your health professional immediately.

- Change in bowel or bladder habits
- A sore that doesn't heal
- Unusual bleeding or discharge

- Thickening or lump in the breast or anywhere on your body
- Indigestion or swallowing difficulty
- Obvious change in a wart or mole
- Nagging cough or hoarseness

Lower Your Risk for Cancer

Cancer is caused by chemicals, radiation, viruses, hormones, immune and metabolic conditions, and inherited gene mutations. While some of these factors are beyond your control, there are many you can do something about. Aging, smoking, and alcohol are the biggest cancer risk factors, and while we can't turn back the clock, we can learn to take better care of ourselves, avoid smoking, and drink moderately. Obesity also raises the risk for certain cancers, as does lack of exercise and poor nutritional status. Dietary risk factors include diets low in fiber and high in fat, smoked foods such as barbecued, pickled foods, and immoderate alcohol usage. Other risk factors include exposure to known carcinogens such as cigarette smoke, radiation (including sunlight), chemicals (including pharmaceutical drugs and pesticides), viruses, and certain parasites. The following guidelines may reduce your risk for cancer.

- Give up tobacco (smoking or chewing).
- Limit your exposure to the sun.
- Use alcohol moderately, if at all.
- Limit radiation and chemical exposure.
- Weigh carefully the benefits and risks of hormone replacement therapy.

- Eat a well-balanced diet emphasizing fresh fruits, vegetables, and lean sources of protein. Diets high in fat, and in smoked and cured foods, may contribute to cancer
- Excessive sugar intake and recreational drugs may also contribute

Professional Treatment

- Nausea, bloating, gas, vomiting: Quiet Digestion (2 tablets three times per day), Chzyme (2 tablets three times per day), and vitamin B$_6$ (100 mg. per day) are helpful. Chewing candied ginger before and after treatments can help relieve chemotherapy-induced nausea. Acupressure wristbands that stimulate an acupuncture point inside the wrist, and regular acupuncture treatments before and during treatments, can also help
- To promote healing after surgery: Resinall K (½ to 1 dropperful under the tongue; hold under tongue until dissolved or applied topically to the skin), Resinall E tablets (3 to 5 tablets three times per day)
- Diarrhea: Colostroplex (1 to 4 tablets per day), Source Qi (4 to 6 tablets three times per day)
- Heat signs due to chemotherapy and radiation: Dandelion tea *(pu gong ying),* Clear Heat (2 to 3 tablets three to four times per day)
- Dryness due to chemotherapy and radiation: Tremella & American Ginseng (3 to 5 tablets four times per day)
- Bone marrow depletion/low blood cell counts: Marrow Plus (3 tablets three to four times per day), Antler 8 (3 tablets three times per day), Astra 8 (3 tablets two to three times per day), Backbone (3 tablets three times per day), gelatin as a food

- Sore throat: Isatis Gold (3 tablets every two to four hours), Cold Away (3 tablets four to six times per day)
- Prevention: Regeneration (2 to 3 tablets three times per day), Power Mushrooms (1 to 3 tablets three times per day), CordySeng (1 to 3 tablets two to three times per day), Bupleurum Entangled Qi (3 tablets three times per day)
- Pain: Channel Flow (2 to 3 tablets three to four times per day)
- Prevent clotting: Resinall E (3 to 5 tablets three times per day), Channel Flow (2 to 3 tablets three to four times per day), EPAQ krill oil (3 soft gel capsules per day with meals)
- Urinary tract infections: Akebia Moist Heat (3 tablets three times per day), Drain Dampness (3 tablets three times per day)
- Fatigue: Chinese tonic herbs can help support and strengthen your body during chemotherapy and radiation treatments. Adrenosen (2 to 3 tablets three times per day), Astra 8 (3 tablets two to three times per day), Power Mushrooms (2 to 3 tablets three times per day), CordySeng (1 to 3 tablets two to three times per day)
- Night sweats: Great Yin (3 tablets three times per day), Nine Flavor Tea (3 tablets three times per day), Tremella & American Ginseng (3 to 5 tablets four times per day)
- Mouth ulcers: Resinall K (½ to 1 dropperful under the tongue; hold under tongue until dissolved), Coptis Purge Fire (3 tablets three times per day), glutamine (3 to 10 g. per day, swish and swallow)
- Mouth sores: Avoid spicy, salty, and acidic foods, which aggravate mouth sores. Sucking on licorice tablets or slippery elm lozenges can soothe mucous membranes. A glutamine mouthwash, made from glutamine powder available at health food stores, can also decrease mouth pain

- Radiation burns: Clear Heat wash, Astra C (2 tablets two to four times per day), creams and lotions containing calendula, aloe gel, and vitamin E cream or oil can all soothe burns. Clear Heat can be made as a tea and applied topically. Tamu Oil can be soothing and regenerate the skin. Seaweed may be consumed as a food
- Lowered immunity: Chinese medicine recommends various mushrooms and other herbs to boost immunity. Milk thistle can protect the liver and kidneys from damage. CordySeng (1 to 3 tablets two to three times per day), Astra 8 (3 tablets two to three times per day), Power Mushrooms (1 to 3 tablets three times per day), Coriolus PS (3 tablets two to four times per day)

Case Studies

Case #1

Reyann, a fifty-eight-year-old female, was diagnosed and treated with surgery and radiation for brain cancer two years ago. Her principal symptom was nausea. Her tongue was pale with a white coat, and her pulse was thin. We recommended Stomach Tabs (2 tablets three times per day) with ginger tea. After two weeks Reyann's nausea was significantly improved. At this point we added Coriolus PS (3 tablets three times per day). It was recommended that she stay on Coriolus PS to tonify her immune system and reduce phlegm. After two months she only used Stomach Tabs when there was damp weather, which seemed to worsen the nausea.

Case #2

Ron was a seventy-two-year-old male diagnosed with a slow-growing prostate tumor with elevated PSA levels. He was treated with radioactive seeds inserted into the skin. His main symptoms were burning with urination, and inability to completely void his urine. His tongue was bright red with a slight dark-yellow coat, and his pulse was elevated. Western tests were negative for bacterial infection.

We recommended Clear Heat (2 tablets four times per day) and Akebia Moist Heat (2 tablets four times per day) to reduce heat, and damp-heat. We also suggested he drink at least 64 oz. of water per day. After two weeks his symptoms were improved, though not eliminated. His tongue was less red and now had a white-yellow thin coat, and his pulse was unchanged. At this point we suggested using the herbs for an additional two weeks. Because there was no longer burning urination, we substituted Essence Chamber (3 tablets three times per day) for Clear Heat. Essence Chamber has saw palmetto and other supportive herbs to help void the urine. After one month his pulse was slower and his tongue was red with a normal white coat. We suggested he stop Akebia Moist Heat. As he was having only slight problems voiding his urine, it was recommended that he take Power Mushrooms (3 tablets three times per day) to fortify his immune system and to drain dampness and that he remain on Essence Chamber (2 tablets three times per day) for the next month. Ron thought the Power Mushrooms improved his energy. We suggested he maintain on this protocol for the next six months.

Case #3

Rusty was a forty-four-year-old detective who was diagnosed with a spinal cord tumor. He had received both surgery and radiation. His symptoms were extreme perianal pain, low back and hip pain, numbness in the feet, difficulty walking, insomnia, and constipation. The only thing that helped the pain was ice packs although he was also prescribed Vicodin for pain. His pulse was irregular, and his tongue was scarlet and dry.

We recommended Formula H (5 tablets three times per day) to reduce heat and swelling in the perianal area, and to indirectly relieve the constipation. We also recommended sitz baths with smilax (2 Tbsp. poured in bathwater) at least twice per day. After two weeks pain was reduced significantly, and his use of Vicodin had decreased. His pulse and tongue were unchanged. At this point we reduced the Formula H to 3 tablets three times per day and added Regeneration (3 tablets three times per day) in order to circulate blood and reduce toxicity. After a month his use of ice packs and Vicodin was reduced by 75 percent. Although he was happy with the results, he could not come in for regular appointments; therefore, we had him maintain on Coriolus PS (3 tablets three times per day) to reduce heat and tonify his immune system and Regeneration (3 tablets three times per day).

Case #4

Mavis was an eighty-six-year-old patient diagnosed with colon cancer that had spread to the lymph nodes. She was brought to the clinic by her grown sons. She had been treated with surgery followed by radiation and chemotherapy. When we saw Mavis, her main symptoms were constipation induced by morphine used to control pain, extreme fatigue, poor appetite, and mouth sores. Her tongue was red and swollen with a dark coating in the rear; her pulse was sinking, thready, and rapid. While the patient was not entirely lucid during the consultation, her sons explained that their hope was not that their mother's cancer could be cured but that we could improve her quality of life. We recommended a traditional tea based on Raise Qi *(bu zhong yi qi tang)* (16 oz. per day), and added Gentle Senna tablets (3 to 6 tablets per day) to promote bowel movement. After two weeks Mavis appeared more lucid. Her sons reported that their mother seemed to have greater energy and improved spirits. Her pulse was stronger, and her tongue was no longer coated. We continued on the same herbs. Two months later one of her sons called to report that his mother had passed on but he wanted to let us know that the herbs had definitely helped improve his mother's quality of life.

Candida Esophagitis

This is an infection of the esophagus caused by candida yeast, and usually occurs in persons with depressed immune systems. Symptoms include inflammation of the esophagus with painful swallowing. Conventional treatment is to use anti-fungal drugs, such as Nizoral. Concurrent herbal therapy can be undertaken by combining Phellostatin (2 to 3 tablets three times per day) and herbal anti-fungals such as Pau D'Arco tea (8 cups per day) and Biocidin (1 to 6 drops with meals).

Case Study

Carl, at thirty-eight, was undergoing chemotherapy and developed Candida esophagitis and thrush, causing difficulty swallowing. He was being treated with Nizoral. Traditional Chinese diagnosis showed that he had a heavy yellow tongue coating and his pulse was sinking and rapid. I recommended Pau D'Arco tea (8 cups per day), Biocidin (3 drops in water, gargled before each meal), and Phellostatin (3 tablets three times per day before meals). After one week the thrush was significantly reduced and he was having an easier time swallowing. His tongue coating was also not as thick.

Candidiasis

According to holistic professionals, candida yeast infection can cause or contribute to all digestive symptoms, and can induce other symptoms such as fatigue, headaches, joint and muscle aches, and menstrual irregularities. Western doctors, on the other hand, feel that candidiasis is only a problem with vaginal yeast infection, thrush, and candida esophagitis.

Normally, healthy intestinal bacteria, the right acid/alkaline balance, and a properly working immune system keep candida, a resident member of our intestinal tract, from getting out of control. However, immune-suppressive drugs such as antibiotics, hormones (including birth control pills), steroids, and chemotherapy can result in yeast overgrowth.

I have found that an anti-yeast diet, as well as dietary supplements and herbs, are very useful. This is especially true if there is a past history of using the above-mentioned drugs (particularly antibiotics), and if there are such accompanying signs as a history of vaginal yeast infections, athlete's foot, jock itch, or fungal infections of the nails or skin. Other indications include symptoms that worsen in damp weather or in moldy buildings, and cravings for sweets and yeast-containing foods (such as beer, wine, bread, and cheese). Although physicians can administer tests to determine if you have excess levels of candida, such tests are often expensive. Furthermore, it is possible to have a sensitivity to normal levels of yeast.

The Digestive Clearing program described in Chapter Four consists of a diet that is free of alcohol, sweets, and yeast-containing foods.

Self-Help

◆ Pau D'Arco tea (6 cups daily) has anti-candida properties and is an excellent beverage for those undergoing anti-candida therapy

◆ Garlic has anti-fungal properties, but should not be used by persons with hot constitutions or with a sensitivity to garlic (dosage is 1 or 2 cloves per day)

◆ Yeast Guard is a homeopathic suppository that can be used

Professional Treatment

◆ Phellostatin is a formula I helped develop and is designed to alter the ecology of the intestines; the formula contains anti-yeast herbs along with digestive tonics. General dosage is 1 tablet three times per day for the first two weeks, and 2 to 3 tablets three times per day thereafter. The therapies listed below may be useful in conjunction, to either assist the digestive system or promote rapid elimination of yeast. By using several natural therapies simultaneously it is possible to achieve comparable results to prescription drugs

◆ Biocidin (use as directed) helps to rapidly kill off yeast; it should be used with Phellostatin or a digestive tonic such as Six Gentlemen because it is very cold in property, and Phellostatin and Six Gentlemen can offset Biocidin's coldness

◆ Aquilaria 22 (1 to 3 tablets three times per day) can be used alone or with Phellostatin in cases of constipation; it has anti-yeast and anti-parasitic properties

◆ Colostroplex (bovine colostrum) (1 to 2 tablets three times per day; reduce dosage if constipation occurs) is used with Phellostatin to improve digestive immunity and to treat diarrhea. Colostroplex has anti-viral and anti-bacterial properties and may have anti-fungal properties as well

◆ Quiet Digestion (2 tablets three times per day) treats food stagnation and acute digestive symptoms

◆ Vagistatin (1 to 2 capsules at bedtime) is an herbal anti-fungal vaginal suppository

Prescription Anti-Fungal Medications

◆ **Nystatin** is an anti-fungal medication that is more than forty years old. It comes in cream, ointment, suppository, tablet, and powder forms. The advantage of the powder form is that it can be used in a gargle, douche, or enema for rapid effect. Nystatin is safe for long-term usage, but follow your physician's dosage recommendations carefully. Symptoms may temporarily worsen when starting any anti-fungal medication—this is known as a die-off reaction. Rebound reactions, in which the yeast infection recurs with severe intensity when the drug is discontinued, also occur, which is why I recommend that Phellostatin herbal formula be taken with these drugs.

◆ **Nizoral (ketoconazole)** is a broad-spectrum anti-fungal drug. Some patients are better able to tolerate Nizoral than Nystatin; however, a small percentage experience liver problems from use of this drug. If you have a history of liver problems, or if you take this drug for more than three months, your liver function should be monitored. Since Nizoral is toxic to the liver, I suggest that Ecliptex herbal formula (2 tablets three times per day) or milk thistle (follow label directions) be taken two weeks for every week on Nizoral.

- **Diflucan (fluconazole)** is more effective than Nizoral at combating yeast infections. It works over a shorter period of time and is not harmful to the liver. Unfortunately, Diflucan is expensive at more than $10 per pill whereas Nizoral costs about $1 to $2 per pill.
- **Sporanox (itraconazole)** appears to be more effective than Nizoral. Some patients may be intolerant to Diflucan, but are better able to tolerate Sporanox and vice versa.

Case Studies

Case #1
A woman was in her late thirties when she came to be treated for PMS, sudden weight gain, fatigue, depression, and abdominal cramping. Her medical doctor, whose diagnosis was candida-related complex, had previously treated her with Diflucan. The client reported that the Diflucan therapy had improved her fatigue and depression by about 50 percent. I suggested that she follow an anti-candida diet, and also recommended she take the formula Woman's Balance (2 tablets four times per day) for the PMS, as well as Unlocking (2 tablets four times per day) for the abdominal cramping. With this protocol, she noticed a definite improvement of her symptoms in three months.

Case #2
Emelio was a forty-five-year-old cook who had numerous health complaints including sinusitis, frequent ear infections, chronic sore throat, frequent and burning urination, fatigue, low back pain, poor sleep, joint pain, tinnitus, hypertension, poor digestion, constipation, and chronic cold hands and feet. He had a history of hepatitis and had been recently diagnosed as having

chronic fatigue syndrome by a holistic medical doctor who placed Emelio on anti-fungal drugs, including Nystatin and Diflucan. He had also prescribed acupuncture, vitamins, and homeopathics. Even though all these remedies had helped, Emelio reported that he was so tired he could "barely make it through the day," and that he still had the above-mentioned complaints.

Traditional Chinese diagnosis found that his pulse was racing and his tongue purplish, with a thick coating on the sides. He had signs of heat in the upper burner and kidney yang deficiency; therefore, the treatment principle was to tonify the yang and remove pathogenic heat and dampness. We recommended that he abstain from alcohol, reduce his intake of sugar, including fruit sugar, and increase his protein intake. Since he admitted to ejaculating several times a day, he was urged to limit this because ejaculation is said to deplete the kidney essence, causing fatigue, low back pain, weak knees, and frequent urination. He was advised to take Coptis Purge Fire (3 tablets four times per day) with Astra Isatis (3 tablets four times per day). During his next visit two weeks later, he reported slightly more energy and less burning with urination. As his pulse was not as excessive, and his face less red, the dosage of Coptis Purge Fire was reduced (2 tablets four times per day), and Shen Gem (2 tablets four times per day) was added, while the dosage of Astra Isatis remained the same.

After one month on the second protocol, Emelio reported feeling more energy and no longer had burning with urination. His pulse was hollow and slightly irregular; his tongue, however, was normal. At this point, Coptis Purge Fire was discontinued, but because fatigue was still a problem, Power Mushrooms was recommended. The new regimen thus consisted of Power Mushrooms (2 tablets four times per day), Astra Isatis (2 tablets four times per day), and Shen Gem (2 tablets four times per day). Emelio noticed some digestive discomfort after starting this protocol and was instructed to reduce the dosage of Power Mushrooms. But he then indicated that he had experienced an increase in energy after starting on the Power Mushrooms, thus elected to stay on the original dosage. Although his treatment protocol varied over the next nine months, most of Emelio's symptoms disappeared through continued herbal therapy.

Case #3

Eleanor, a graphic designer in her early forties, complained of severe PMS, weight gain, chronic fatigue, fibromyalgia, and depression. A battery of tests taken at Stanford University was inconclusive. She visited an M.D. specializing in chronic fatigue syndrome, who placed her on a trial therapy of the anti-fungal medication Diflucan, which appeared to improve her symptoms by about 50 percent. She sought additional relief at our clinic.

Eleanor's initial traditional Chinese syndrome pattern was one of damp-heat, primarily of dampness, which was manifested by symptoms of overweight and worsening of joint and muscle pain in rainy weather or damp environments. Her pulse was slippery, and her tongue had a grayish yellow coating. Based on her pattern presentation and the fact that she was benefiting from the Diflucan, and that she had been on several courses of antibiotics each year during the past decade to treat cystitis and bronchial infections—additional indicators of damp-heat—we decided to start her on an anti-candida diet that eliminated alcohol, sweets, and yeast-containing foods. We also suggested two herbal formulas, Phellostatin (1 tablet three times per day the first week, 2 tablets three times per day thereafter) and Woman's Balance (2 tablets three times per day), as well as Astra Diet Tea, to be consumed several times throughout the day as a substitute for sweets, and to promote energy and reduce phlegm.

Eleanor had great trouble adhering to the recommended diet so it was not surprising that after three weeks she had noticed little change in her symptoms. We encouraged her to do her best, stressing that if she stopped her nightly wine consumption she would in all likelihood feel better and even lose weight. Nevertheless, she did notice less fluid retention during her first premenstrual phase since coming to our clinic, but the mood swings and irritability remained. Six weeks after starting the herbal formulas and following the diet as best as she could, she finally reduced her wine intake to Saturday nights only. She had also lost 5 pounds and felt more clear headed. During her second premenstrual phase, she noticed significantly fewer mood swings, less irritability, and less fluid retention. By her third period, nearly all PMS symptoms were resolved. At this time, we recommended that she stay on the Woman's Balance premenstrually, and take Phellostatin (same dosage) and Aspiration (3 tablets three times per day). The latter was used to relieve depression as it contains specific herbs such as vervain, polygala *(yuan zhi),* and albizzia *(he huan hua)* for that purpose.

Case #4
William was a thirty-year-old sales representative who complained of fatigue, athlete's foot, and chronic intestinal gas. He was away from home two to three weeks every month, and undoubtedly his constant restaurant eating was a major contributing factor to his digestive disorders. In addition, after his daily meetings and sales calls, he usually had several alcoholic beverages; and when he was home, he typically smoked marijuana to relax. Traditional Chinese diagnosis revealed that his pulse was slow, sinking, and slightly wiry, and his tongue was red with a thick, greasy yellow coating. I recommended Phellostatin (2 tablets three times per day) to tonify the spleen, clear heat, and rid the body of fungus. He was also given Quiet Digestion (2 tablets three times per day) since it possesses herbs that address flatulence, resolve dampness, and relieve food stagnation,

which causes intestinal gas. I also suggested 2 capsules of PB8 acidophilus to be taken at bedtime.

In terms of dietary and lifestyle habits, he was advised to reduce or eliminate alcohol, which promotes the growth of yeast, and to reduce or stop his marijuana use, which through its laxative effects will over time weaken the spleen and lead to accumulation of dampness. Furthermore, fungal mold is known to contaminate marijuana. I also recommended low sugar and non-fermented foods, and gave him a supplemental list of foods that can cause gas such as beans, peas, wheat, oats, bran, brussels sprouts, cabbage, corn, rutabaga, and dairy products.

At his next visit one month later, William reported that the symptoms of gas were reduced by about 50 percent and that his energy level had increased slightly. But he also expressed his disappointment that his condition was not cured. His pulse was thin and wiry, and although his tongue no longer had a thick coating, it was now pale in the center and red on the edges. I asked him if he had made any of the recommended dietary and lifestyle changes, to which he replied that because he traveled so often, it was difficult—if not impossible—to change his habits while on the road. I pointed out that if he wanted to "cure" his intestinal gas he would have to make the dietary changes, and suggested that he locate health food stores and perhaps restaurants that serve healthy cuisines in the cities he visited instead of going to standard restaurants. I also indicated that he should get more exercise. With regard to his herbal therapy, I recommended that he finish the bottle of Phellostatin that he had (2 tablets three times per day), remain on Quiet Digestion (2 tablets as needed) and PB8 (2 capsules at bedtime), and add Ecliptex (2 tablets three times per day) to soothe the liver.

By his next visit a month later he had reduced his alcohol intake to one drink per night. He indicated that the problem with gas remained about the same, but Quiet Digestion proved symptomatically effective. He also reported that he had developed insomnia and acid reflux, which he first tried to blame on his reduction in alcohol, but later admitted he was having marital problems largely as a result of being away from home so long. William's pulse remained wiry and his tongue unchanged. At this point, I added Ease Plus (2 tablets four times per day) to his treatment plan, in order to calm the nerves, spread liver qi, and reduce stomach acidity. Quiet Digestion and PB8 were continued at the same dosages.

Discussion: The herbs appeared to be helpful, but did not resolve William's condition. This was because of his excessive traveling in addition to marital problems, both of which created stress such that he relied on alcohol for relief.

Cat Scratch Fever

Cat Scratch Fever is an infection generally thought to be contracted from a cat's scratch, bite, or lick. Symptoms appear several days after contact with a cat, and include swollen, painful lymph nodes, achiness, loss of appetite, headache, fever, and fatigue. Although most cases subside without treatment after a few weeks, antibiotics may speed recovery, particularly in people with compromised immune systems.[6]

Professional Treatment

- ◆ Reduce fever: Clear Heat (2 to 3 tablets three to four times per day) or can be made into a tea and applied as a wash topically: to cool affected area crush 2 tablets and add to boiling water, steep for fifteen minutes, strain, and apply with washcloth

◆ Poor appetite: Chzyme (2 tablets two to three times per day)

Chickenpox

Chickenpox is caused by the varicella-zoster virus, which spreads through the air and physical contact. The signature symptom of chickenpox is an itchy, red rash on the face, chest, and back. The rash appears within two weeks of exposure, starting as spots that turn into blisters that break open and crust over. Prior to the appearance of the rash, there may also be fever, runny nose, dry cough, irritability, fatigue, weakness, and mild headache. People with chickenpox are contagious about forty-eight hours before the appearance of the rash, until all spots have crusted over.

A vaccine called Varivax became available in 1995, and today children are routinely immunized for chickenpox. Also, once you've had chickenpox, you're usually immune for life. While chickenpox usually passes in about two weeks without complications in healthy children, it can cause serious complications including pneumonia and encephalitis in adults, infants, teenagers, and people with suppressed immune function. Doctors may prescribe an anti-viral drug such as acyclovir (Zovirax) for these high-risk groups. In uncomplicated cases, a visit to the doctor isn't usually necessary, but it's time to call the doctor if the rash involves the eye, gets very red, warm, and tender (indicating a skin infection), or is accompanied by a fever higher than 103°F, dizziness, disorientation, rapid heartbeat, shortness of breath, tremors, loss of muscle coordination, worsening cough, vomiting, or stiff neck.

About one in five adults who had chickenpox as children will have shingles later in life, usually after age fifty. In shingles, the varicella-zoster virus reactivates, causing a painful band of blisters.

When pain persists after the blisters are gone, it's called postherpetic neuralgia.[7]

Self-Help

Self-care for mild cases of chickenpox includes:

- To ease itching: calamine lotion, baths with uncooked oatmeal or baking soda
- To reduce fever: lukewarm baths and acetaminophen (Tylenol). Do not use aspirin with chickenpox because it's associated with a serious condition called Reye's syndrome, which causes swelling of the brain and liver dysfunction, and can lead to brain damage and coma.

Professional Treatment

- To reduce fever: Clear Heat (2 to 3 tablets three to four times per day) or can be made into a tea and applied as a wash topically: to cool affected area crush 2 tablets and add to boiling water, steep for fifteen minutes, strain, and apply with washcloth

Case Study

Kelly was a sixty-two-year-old female diagnosed with postherpetic neuralgia. Her main symptoms were a constant burning pain in the chest area, depression, and fatigue. Kelly was prescribed Vicodin and Zovirax by her HMO. Kelly's pulse was wiry; her tongue was pale with red spots. We suggested Resinall K topically over the affected area three to six times per day and orally

(½ dropperful three times per day) with Channel Flow (2 tablets three times per day). Both Resinall K and Channel Flow have pain-relieving properties. After two weeks Kelly was able to experience a slight reduction in pain and had reduced her Vicodin usage by 50 percent. Her tongue was unchanged and her pulse was less wiry. After two more weeks Kelly was able to decrease her Vicodin use further and reported a modest reduction in pain. As her pain was reduced she reported being able to go out of the house more frequently, and this improved her mood. After six weeks, she only occasionally needed the Vicodin, and reported her pain 80 percent reduced. Her tongue was normal colored with dots, and her pulse was improved. At this point we had her take Astra Isatis (3 tablets three times per day) to attack the virus and to strengthen her immune system. She maintained on Resinall K topically and internally.

Chronic Fatigue Syndrome (CFS)

Fatigue is ubiquitous in our culture today, and particularly plagues people with immune system issues. Chronic fatigue syndrome is also called chronic fatigue immune dysfunction syndrome (CFIDS). Studies show that people with chronic fatigue syndrome and fibromyalgia often have immune system dysfunctions that can result in unusual infections such as HHV-6, CMV, EBV, parasites, mycoplasma, chlamydia, Lyme disease, and most importantly, fungal/yeast infections. These tips for alleviating fatigue are designed to be useful for readers diagnosed with CFS and other conditions in which fatigue is a primary symptom, as well as for those of us who are just plain tired.

Chronic fatigue syndrome was originally named following a 1984 outbreak in Incline Village, Nevada, though medical practitioners have observed similar syndromes for more than a century.

For example, back in the late 1800s, women were commonly diagnosed with *neurasthenia,* which shared many symptoms with CFS, including "nervous exhaustion." More commonly diagnosed in women than in men, CFS is an umbrella term for illness characterized by the sudden onset of extreme, debilitating fatigue, muscle and joint pain, tender lymph nodes, headaches, and poor concentration. For many people, symptoms set in after an illness, such as a cold, intestinal bug, or mononucleosis, or during a stressful time in their life. Unlike flu symptoms, these symptoms hang on, or come and go, for months. In the 1980s, laboratory tests led scientists to speculate that CFS was related to the Epstein-Barr virus, but while many people with CFS symptoms test positive for this virus, many also show no signs of it.

Because the symptoms of CFS resemble so many other diseases and syndromes—including fibromyalgia, multiple sclerosis, and systemic lupus erythematosus—CFS can be difficult to diagnose. Generally, exhaustion for six months or more, and at least four of the following diagnostic criteria, merit a positive diagnosis for CFS: sore throat, painful lymph nodes in the neck or armpits, headaches, unexplained muscle soreness, migrating pain without redness or swelling, impaired memory and concentration, insomnia, inability to tolerate exercise that was once tolerable, and irritable bowel syndrome.

Fibromyalgia is another condition that usually comes with fatigue, and often looks very much like CFS. Fibromyalgia is characterized by muscle pain throughout the body, and is diagnosed by tenderness at eleven of eighteen characteristic locations on the neck, upper back, rib cage, hips, and knees. Associated symptoms include fatigue, stiffness, insomnia, anxiety, depression, mood swings, allergies, and carpal tunnel syndrome, as well as Raynaud's phenomenon and irritable bowel syndrome. Like chronic fatigue syndrome, fibromyalgia is difficult to diagnose because its symptoms resemble many other

214

disorders. Diagnosis involves many tests to rule out other conditions. Symptoms may be controlled with moderate exercise and physical therapy, reducing stress, and improving sleep, along with complementary therapies such as acupuncture, massage, and relaxation techniques. Doctors may prescribe sleep aids and analgesics, along with an antidepressant, many of which help with sleep.[8]

Health experts recommend a balanced diet, adequate rest, moderate exercise, and counseling to cope with the difficult emotions associated with the uncertainty of the condition. NSAIDs like ibuprofen can alleviate aches and fever.

Self-Help

Getting seven to nine hours of good sleep a night is key to fighting fatigue, but getting good sleep is not always as easy as it seems. If you're having a hard time sleeping, see the "Insomnia" section later in this chapter. Patients who eat a lot of processed food may develop nutritional deficiencies. Bowel infections can also make it harder for your body to absorb nutrients, just when illness is making your body hungry for extra nutrients. Here's a short list of the most important nutrients for people dealing with CFS.

- Arginine (2 to 3 g. per day) stimulates growth hormone. Do not use if you have herpes
- Colostrum contains IgF-1, which fights infections and may potentiate growth hormone
- Adrenal cortex extract
- Avoid sweets—use stevia instead
- Take probiotics (use as directed) to balance microflora

- Garlic (1 to 3 cloves a day) in olive oil or yogurt for yeast or parasitic infections
- Oregano oil (1 capsule two to three times per day)
- Adequate protein—it's important to consume protein with every meal, in the form of eggs, lean meat, poultry, and protein shakes
- Antioxidants, B vitamins, B12, NAC (N-acetylcysteine) 500 to 1,000 mg. per day, which increases glutathione
- Iron (for those with anemia), magnesium, and selenium (200 mcg. per day to reduce infections)
- Essential fatty acids, from flax or fish oils (200 to 800 mg. per day)
- Shiitake soup—1 to 3 buttons, simmer in water for 15 minutes
- L-Carnitine (2 to 10 g. per day)

Professional Treatment

- Astra Isatis (2 tablets four times per day) or Astra 8 (if no signs of heat or lymphatic swelling); combine Astra Isatis or Astra 8 with Power Mushrooms (2 tablets four times per day)
- Phellostatin (2 to 3 tablets three times per day) if candida or fungus
- Adrenosen (2 tablets three times per day) to restore energy levels; does not contain stimulants
- Channel Flow (2 to 3 tablets three times per day) for pain and stiffness

Case Studies

Case #1

Roland was diagnosed with chronic fatigue syndrome three years ago after a stressful divorce and getting laid off. His main symptoms were exhaustion and difficulty concentrating, arm and leg cramping and spasms. He was currently taking trazodone to help him sleep. He was also under the care of a chiropractor who recommended several enzyme products and an anti-candida formula. Roland's tongue was pale and wet; his pulse was slow. Our first recommendation was that Roland stop taking the anti-candida formula as it contained a number of ingredients that were too energetically cold for his constitution. We also suggested that he simplify the number of enzymes he was taking as there seemed to be an overlap in the products.

We recommended Astra Essence (3 tablets three times per day) to tonify Qi, blood, and kidneys; and SPZM (3 tablets three times per day) to relax his tendons and to reduce cramping; and cinnamon tea to warm his body. After two weeks there was a modest improvement in Roland's energy level, and a slight reduction in cramping. Over time Roland's energy increased substantially, his ability to concentrate improved, and the leg and arm cramps were reduced.

Case # 2

Delores was an overweight sixty-four-year-old retired teacher with exhaustion as her main symptom and muscle and joint pain as secondary symptoms. Delores woke up tired after eight to ten hours of sleep, and said she needed one to two naps just to make it through the day. Slight exercise such as swimming or walking often provoked extreme fatigue and pain. Delores was taking the medications Provigil (modafinil), which increases dopamine and is used to improve wakefulness; Wellbutrin (bupropion HCl); and ibuprofen for pain. Her tongue was swollen and pale, and her pulse wiry in the liver position and sinking in all other positions. We recommended Ease 2 (3 tablets three times per day) in order to spread liver qi and tonify the spleen, and Adrenosen, in an herbal formula to promote adrenal function and reduce fatigue (2 tablets three times per day). We suggested walking and abdominal massage twenty minutes per day, and protein with each meal.

Delores was not able to come for follow-up until three weeks later. During this time she had to go to a large family gathering, which lasted all weekend and involved a long drive. Although her husband commented that Delores seemed to have more energy and more reserves during the family gathering, Delores said she felt about the same. She did not comply with the abdominal massage recommendation. Her pulse was weak but less wiry in the liver position and slightly stronger overall. Her tongue was slightly less swollen, though still pale. We suggested she add EPAQ krill oil (3 soft gel capsules per day with meals) to reduce inflammation and for its energizing effects. After two weeks Delores' energy had improved dramatically. Her pulse was stronger and her tongue was less pale though still swollen. Her new protocol was Six Gentlemen to tonify the spleen and reduce dampness (3 tablets three times per day), Adrenosen (2 tablets three times per day), and EPAQ krill oil (3 soft gel capsules per day with meals). Ease 2 was eliminated as her pulse was no longer wiry and her pain was reduced.

Case #3 Candida overtreatment

Lois was a sixty-five-year-old, overweight homemaker whose chief complaints were fatigue, muscle and joint pain, and easy bruising. Her chiropractor had recommended an aggressive anti-candida and supplement program that did not seem to be helping, although the diet initially had helped her lose weight. She

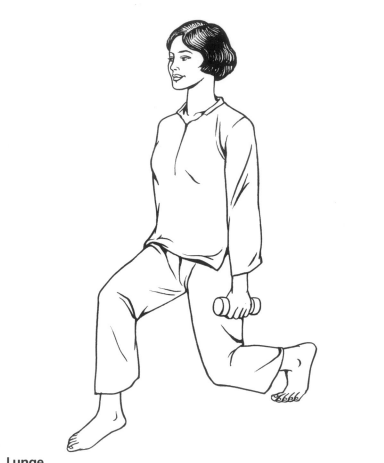

Lunge

Stand with your feet shoulder-width apart and your arms at your sides with a weight in each hand. Take a large step forward with your right foot and lift your left heel so you're up on your left toes. Your right knee should be bent and directly above your right ankle; do not allow your knee to pass your ankle. Press your shoulder back and lift your chin as you slowly lower your left knee toward the floor. Pause when your left knee is as low as it can go, then slowly rise back up, keeping your feet in the same position. Do 12–15 repetitions per set, on each side, completing three sets. *Precaution:* Try not to dip too low if your knees are weak.

was currently taking caprylic acid capsules, oregano drops, and Pau D'Arco tincture for candida. In addition, she took glucosamine and chondroitin capsules, and ibuprofen for pain. Lois was pale, her pulse was thin, slow, and sinking, and her tongue were pale with a heavy white coat.

Our first suggestion was that she eliminate the anti-candida supplements. In our experience these substances can be overly cooling and in some cases ineffective at the dose that is administered. We recommended Adrenosen (2 tablets three times per day) to bolster the adrenals and to increase her energy, and Marrow Plus (3 tablets three times per day) to nourish her blood. We suggested taking the herbs with ginger tea (3 cups per day), which improves digestive function and can reduce pain.

After two weeks, Lois reported that she felt more energetic, but the pain was unchanged. Her pulse felt more robust, and her tongue showed reduced coating. After one month her fatigue was markedly better and her joint and muscle pain slightly improved. At this point we added SAMe (2 tablets two times per day) to help with her joint and muscle pain and also the fatigue.

After three months Lois had plenty of energy, and felt that her pain was greatly reduced, although sometimes she woke up stiff or had pain when she worked in her garden too much.

Discussion: Anti-candida programs can be very beneficial particularly for people who have digestive problems, and unexplained symptoms such as joint and muscle pain. As a strict anti-candida diet includes no sweetened foods or beverages, and low amounts of starchy food, it typically will assist in weight loss. As Lois appeared to be blood deficient, it appeared that her joint and muscle pain was due to aging and the fact that she was overweight, which puts pressure on the joints. As it was making her body colder, I thought it was best to discontinue the anti-candida supplements. SAMe is useful to treat joint and muscle pain, and many clients find it energizing.

Common Cold and Flu

The common cold is a mild viral respiratory infection. Other viral respiratory illnesses include laryngitis, pharyngitis, bronchitis, croup, and pneumonia. Cold symptoms include a watery, runny nose that becomes congested, sneezing, watery eyes, sore throat, hoarseness, cough, slight fever, body aches, chills, headache, and fatigue. Colds are more common in children, as part of their immune system's learning process, and in individuals with a weak immune system. Colds are spread by contact with an infected person. The onset of a cold usually occurs one to two days after exposure and may be signaled by an itching or sore throat, or a watery, runny nose, with other symptoms appearing later. With more than two hundred different viral strains that can cause a cold, symptoms can vary considerably. Because colds are caused by viruses, they should not be treated with antibiotics. See a health professional if your fever is high, or your symptoms are severe or have lasted more than ten days. Usually it is best to rest and drink plenty of fluids. Biomedical options include taking aspirin or ibuprofen for pain, along with the self-help strategies listed below.

Symptoms of influenza, or flu, are similar to symptoms of the common cold, but flu symptoms are more severe. Flu is typically spread between people indoors, and its symptoms come on suddenly. These symptoms include fever and chills, sore throat, cough, muscle pain, fatigue, and congestion. Technically, there are three types of influenza, although laypeople often refer to other viral infections as the flu. Physicians may diagnosis influenza by a throat culture or blood test, which may be important if you have a particularly strong flu, if your doctor suspects pneumonia or a bacterial infection. Biomedical solutions include rest, drinking plenty of fluids, and taking analgesics or cough medicine. The anti-viral drug amantadine is administered if you have influenza type A, the type usually responsible for influenza epidemics. Physicians also recommend vaccines for seniors and those with a weak immune system.

Self-Help

- Gargle with salt water (½ tsp. to a large glass of water). It is helpful to alternate with fresh lemon juice (the juice of 1 lemon per large glass of water)
- Look for products in tablets or capsules containing echinacea and goldenseal (use as directed)
- Take slippery elm for dry cough and hoarseness, 1 tsp. added to 8 oz. boiling water (three times per day)

Professional Treatment

- Isatis Gold (3 tablets every two to three hours), a strong anti-viral and anti-bacterial formula
- Cold Away (3 tablets four to six times per day, between meals); use at the first stages of cold or flu
- Ease 2 (2 tablets four times per day) plus Power Mushrooms (2 tablets four times per day) are used for prolonged colds and flu lasting more than five days

Case Studies

Case #1
Mina was a thirty-six-year-old accountant who complained of fatigue and frequent colds over the past year. Her pulse was deep

and slow, and her tongue purple blue with a heavy white coat. We recommended Astra C (2 tablets three times per day) and Six Gentlemen (3 tablets three times per day). Astra C, which contains the traditional Jade Screen formula with zinc, is used to prevent colds and allergy symptoms. Six Gentlemen was selected to tonify her spleen and eliminate dampness and phlegm. After one month she felt slightly better, her pulse was slightly better, and her tongue had lost some of the coating; therefore, we suggested she stay on the protocol. Over time her protocol was changed to Astra C and Virility Tabs, as she no longer needed the phlegm-clearing effects of Six Gentlemen. Virility Tabs is a strong kidney yang tonic. She stayed on the protocol for six months, with noticeably fewer colds than the previous year.

Case #2

Shelly was a thirty-two-year-old administrative assistant who acquired a staph infection from a hospital stay. Six months later, she was still complaining of constant sinus and urinary tract infections. As a result she had been on antibiotics continuously. Shelly's tongue was pale and swollen with a thin white coating, and her pulse was thin. We recommended Power Mushrooms (3 tablets three times per day) and CordySeng (2 tablets three times per day) to strongly tonify the immune system. In addition, PB8 acidophilus was recommend (4 capsules per day) to replenish healthy bacteria that gets eliminated by antibiotics.

After two weeks Shelly felt much better. After discussing it with her doctor, she decided to stop taking the antibiotics. Her tongue was less swollen, and her pulse was unchanged. She continued on the herbs. After four weeks she felt she was getting a sinus infection. Her pulse was floating and fast, and her tongue was red and dry. We recommended Isatis Gold, and suggested irrigating her sinus with saline and 1 to 3 drops of goldenseal up to six times per day. She maintained on the acidophilus. After a few days, Shelly reported that she no longer felt sick, and returned to the CordySeng and Power Mushrooms. After three weeks, she reported that she felt a sinus infection coming on again. Shelly repeated our previous recommendations, and after two days reported she felt much better. She returned to taking the Power Mushrooms and CordySeng. Shelly stayed on the herbs for six months. Although she did get one sinus infection, which required antibiotics and was not treatable with herbs, her overall health and energy had improved and she no longer needed to take antibiotics every day.

Crohn's Disease and Ulcerative Colitis

Crohn's disease and ulcerative colitis are classifications of inflammatory bowel disease (IBD). They are similar conditions, except that ulcerative colitis occurs in the colon and the rectum, while Crohn's disease, also called regional enteritis, affects any segment of the alimentary canal, from the mouth to the anus. More commonly Crohn's disease involves the last part of the small intestine called the ileum. Mild cases of both diseases can cause such symptoms as intestinal cramping and diarrhea. Severe cases can involve bloody diarrhea, bowel obstruction, fever, weight loss, and in the case of Crohn's disease, joint pain and inflammation in other areas of the body. Diagnosis of either condition is confirmed by barium X-rays, colonoscopy, and biopsy. Conventional treatment consists of medications, including antibiotics and immunosuppressive drugs, as well as corticosteroids, azulfaidine, Asacol, metronidazole (Flagyl), and chemotherapy drugs. Surgery may be required for bowel obstruction or chronic abscesses, but rates of recurrence after surgery are high.

Either form of inflammatory bowel disease is associated with an increased risk of colon cancer. Parasitic infections can mimic

IBD, and I believe those with IBD are more prone to contracting such infections. If parasites are either the cause or a complication, they must be treated first (see "Parasites," later in this chapter).

Crohn's Disease and Food

At the Addenbrooke's Hospital in Cambridge, England, British doctors have successfully treated active Crohn's disease by determining which foods trigger a flare-up, and then eliminating them from the diet. According to Dr. John O. Hunter, this regimen has worked just as well as surgery and drugs. "Patients who develop a satisfactory diet have overall relapse rates of less than ten per year, which matches the success of surgery." According to Dr. Hunter, "diet is more successful than medication. Foods most likely to induce flare-ups are wheat, dairy products, cruciferous vegetables, corn, yeast, tomatoes, citrus fruits, and eggs."[9]

Professional Treatment

- The formula Isatis Cooling (3 to 5 tablets three times per day) and Colostroplex (1 to 3 tablets three times per day) have been used with success. Add Quiet Digestion (1 to 2 tablets with each meal) to help assimilate food
- For stabbing pain and inflammation, use Isatis Cooling alone
- For diarrhea, use Source Qi (3 to 5 tablets three times per day) combined with Colostroplex (1 to 3 tablets three times per day)

- For diarrhea and inflammation, use Phellostatin (1 to 3 tablets three times per day) and Colostroplex (1 to 3 tablets three times per day)
- For bloody stools, administer Formula H (3 to 5 tablets three times per day) and Colostroplex (1 to 3 tablets three times per day)
- Six Gentlemen (3 tablets three times per day) and Astra Essence (3 tablets three times per day) are good follow-up formulas for tonifying and strengthening the body when symptoms have been eliminated

Ear Infection (Otitis Media)

Acute ear infection is characterized by earache, fullness in the ear, hearing loss, fever and chills, nausea, and diarrhea. There are four basic types of ear infection: serous otitis media, otitis media with effusion, purulent otitis media, and secretory otitis media.

With serous otitis media, fluid accumulates in the middle ear as a result of fluid in the ear or a blockage in the eustachian tube. In otitis media with effusion, there is both fluid buildup and infection. This form can lead to the more serious acute purulent otitis media, where pus fills the middle ear. The pressure of the pus may burst the eardrum, resulting in a discharge of blood and pus. Acute purulent otitis media, which mostly affects children, may be caused by either a viral or a bacterial infection. Prolonged episodes of otitis media may change the lining of the inner ear, producing thicker fluids and secretory otitis media.

See your health professional if you have sharp pain that does not let up, hearing loss, and fever. If fluid or pus is visible, a culture should be taken to determine if antibiotics are warranted. Conventional biomedical treatments include using analgesics such as aspirin or ibuprofen, decongestants, and antihistamines. In some cases, surgery is necessary to relieve the pressure in the inner ear.

Chronic ear infection is characterized by prolonged earache, pus draining from the ear, and hearing loss. It may be due to swelling or inflammation of the adenoids in the back of the nasal passage, causing a block in the eustachian tube. Diagnosis is made on the basis of an ear exam, X-ray, or CT scan. Treatment options are similar to those for acute ear infection, with the additional possibility of inserting an ear tube to allow the middle ear to drain.

Self-Help

♦ Food allergy elimination, especially dairy products (see Chapter Four, "Digestive Clearing Diet")
♦ Probiotics (use as directed)
♦ Tea tree oil ear drops (use as directed)

Professional Treatment

♦ Coptis Purge Fire (2 to 3 tablets three to four times per day) used to reduce heat and excessive fluid. Often combined with Nasal Tabs 2 (2 tablets three to four times per day) to reduce congestion and promote draining of fluids
♦ Flavonex (3 tablets three times per day) used for chronic ear infections, to increase circulation and speed healing

Guillain-Barré Syndrome

Guillain-Barré syndrome is a rare autoimmune condition in which the immune system attacks the myelin sheath that surrounds nerves and speeds peripheral nerve signals to the brain. It often occurs a few days or weeks following a respiratory or gastrointestinal infection. The symptoms of Guillain-Barré come on suddenly, starting with feelings of weakness and tingling in the legs, which worsen and spread to the arms and upper body, usually leading to severe though temporary paralysis within two weeks. Knee reflexes are usually lost, and because nerve signals slow, a nerve conduction velocity test can help a doctor diagnose the syndrome. The cerebrospinal fluid contains more protein than normal in Guillain-Barré, so doctors may also order a spinal tap.

In extreme cases, a patient may be placed on a respirator, a heart monitor, or machines that support body functions while the nervous system recovers. Two types of therapy seem to lessen severity of symptoms and speed recovery: plasmapheresis and high-dose immunoglobulin therapy. It's thought that the blood plasma contains the antibodies that are attacking the myelin sheath, and in plasmapheresis, blood is removed from the body, the red and white blood cells separated from the plasma, and those cells then returned to the body, without the plasma. High-dose immunoglobulin therapy involves intravenous injections of properly functioning immunoglobulins, which the immune system used to attack invading organisms. Physical therapy is indicated when limb control returns. Because sudden paralysis can be devastating emotionally, psychological counseling can be helpful.[10]

Professional Treatment

- EPAQ krill oil (3 soft gel capsules daily with meals) to reduce inflammation
- Folic acid (800 mcg. daily) is needed for proper nerve transmission
- Marrow Plus (3 tablets three times per day) treats numbness due to blood deficiency

Headaches

Headache may be caused by an immune disorder, or it may be related to a common culprit such as stress. The three main types of headaches are **tension headaches,** which produce a dull or intense pain over the top of the head or back of the neck; **migraines,** which are characterized by intense head pain accompanied by nausea, vomiting, and visual disturbances, such as seeing auras, rainbows, or blank spots in your vision; and **cluster headaches,** which typically produce a boring, burning pain, frequently around one eye and temple, or the cheek or jaw. Analgesics, steroids, calcium channel blockers, ergot, barbiturates, or sumatriptan may be prescribed.

Headaches may be eased with stress reduction and exercise. For example, biofeedback, acupuncture, tai chi, and yoga can be especially beneficial. A comprehensive program may include evaluation of food allergies or sensitivities, chemical toxicity, and adrenal status.

Self-Help

- Magnesium (200 to 800 mg. per day)

◆ Butterbur root reduces the intensity and duration of migraine attacks, and over time, reduces the number of migraines (50 mg. of lipophilic extract two times per day)

◆ Ginkgo reduces platelet aggregation, and thus improves circulation, to prevent headaches (160 to 240 mg. per day of 24 percent flavonoids)

Professional Treatment

◆ Ease Plus (2 to 4 tablets three times per day) is typically used for chronic headaches worsened by stress

◆ Head Q (3 to 5 tablets three times per day) with feverfew increases circulation and may be symptomatically effective for a wide range of headaches; can be combined with Ease Plus (above)

◆ Glutathione (1 tsp. as needed) is an empirical treatment for headaches

Hodgkin's Disease (Lymphoma) and Non-Hodgkin's Lymphomas

Lymphomas are cancers of the lymphatic system. Hodgkin's disease, named for the doctor who first recognized it in 1832, is a type of lymphoma. It is usually detected following an enlarged lymph node in the neck, armpit, or groin. Lymph nodes may also be enlarged in a variety of conditions, from relatively mild infections to more serious conditions like non-Hodgkin's lymphoma, and other cancers and infectious diseases. Other symptoms may include fever, weight loss, night sweats, and itchy skin. Hodgkin's disease is most likely to affect people between the ages of fifteen and thirty-four, or individuals over sixty, and is more common in males. While the cause of Hodgkin's lymphoma is unknown, some experts suspect a relationship with Epstein-Barr virus, though Hodgkin's is not contagious. Physicians typically diagnose Hodgkin's on the basis of biopsy and blood tests. Radiation and chemotherapy are very effective, particularly if the Hodgkin's is diagnosed in the early stages.

Non-Hodgkin's lymphomas are distinguished from Hodgkin's disease by the absence of a specific type of cell—Reed-Sternberg cells—which are present in lymph tissue with Hodgkin's disease. Non-Hodgkin's lymphomas are more likely to attack the bone marrow, digestive tract, and the skin. In children, the most common early symptoms are anemia, rashes, fatigue, and neurological symptoms, rather than enlarged lymph nodes. Biopsies, CT scans, blood tests, and other screenings are used to diagnose non-Hodgkin's lymphoma. Standard treatments involve radiation, chemotherapy, and bone marrow transplants. Experimental therapies include monoclonal antibodies used to attack the lymphoma cells. Herbal treatments can be designed to support the biomedical treatments.

Professional Treatment

- ◆ Clear Heat (3 tablets three times per day) can be used to reduce lymphatic swelling
- ◆ Formula V (3 tablets two times per day) contains herbs used to reduce swelling, such as lymph edema, and improve circulation.
- ◆ Marrow Plus (3 tablets three times per day) to build blood
- ◆ See "Cancer" section of this chapter

Case Studies

Case #1

Lilly was a fifty-eight-year-old woman, with a history of breast cancer, currently dealing with Hodgkin's disease. In addition to surgery, she was given radiotherapy a few months before the consultation. Her main symptoms were afternoon and night fevers, night sweats, and joint pain. Lilly was on a regimen of antioxidant vitamins, Co Q-10, and calcium D-glucarate. Her tongue was red and dry; her pulse was floating and fast. As all her symptoms indicated yin deficiency with heat, we recommended Great Yin (3 tablets three times per day). After three weeks Lilly had a substantial reduction in the amount of night sweats and fevers. She said her joints felt better but still ached at night. Her tongue was less red, and her pulse was more rooted. At this point we suggested she remain on Great Yin (2 tablets four times per day) and added Mobility 2 (2 tablets four times per day) in order to reduce her joint pain. After one month all her symptoms were resolved, except the joint pain was still present; however, it was being controlled with Advil. As she wanted to fortify her immune system, we recommended Coriolus PS (3 tablets three times per day) as it has some heat-clearing properties and also Astra Essence (2 tablets four times per day) long term. Lilly feels that the herbs and vitamins are helping to improve the functioning of her immune system.

Case #2

Steve was a thirty-nine-year-old male who had completed both radiation and chemotherapy for Hodgkin's lymphoma. As a result, his immune system was weakened and he had contracted pneumonia, which required hospitalization. He was currently on oral antibiotics. His symptoms were shortness of breath, exhaustion, productive cough especially in the morning and a dry cough at night, dizziness, and some indigestion. He was running a low-grade fever in the afternoon and felt cold on the outside and hot on the inside. His pulse was floating and weak; his tongue was red with geographic coating that appeared gray. We recommended Ease 2 (5 tablets three times per day) to treat indigestion, fatigue, and phlegm and CordySeng (2 tablets three times per day) to improve his breathing, reduce his cough, and tonify his immune system. After one week there was a slight improvement in his exhaustion, breathing, and indigestion. His pulse was sinking, thin, and weak; his tongue was red. At this point we substituted Marrow Plus (3 tablets three times per day), a strong blood-building formula, for Ease 2. Marrow Plus was targeted toward reducing the sensation of cold exterior and warm interior and the dizziness. He maintained on the CordySeng. After one month Steve was feeling better, though still tired. His pulse was slightly stronger, and his tongue was unchanged. He maintained on the herbs for several more months.

Human Immunodeficiency Virus (HIV)

HIV is a viral infection that destroys white blood cells, leading to other diseases including AIDS. The virus is spread through sex or contaminated needles, or transferred from a mother to her unborn child via the bloodstream. Exposure to HIV does not always lead to infection, and many infected people remain well for more than a decade after the initial infection. People with HIV may be asymptomatic, or may begin to notice fatigue, fever, rashes, and swollen lymph nodes in the beginning stages. Other symptoms that may develop over time include weight loss, diarrhea, anemia, and thrush. As the lymphocyte count begins to drop, opportunistic infections and cancers such as Kaposi's sarcoma and non-Hodgkin's lymphoma may develop. Common opportunistic infections include pneumonia, tuberculosis, mycobacterium avium, cytomegalovirus, toxoplasmosis, and cryptosporidium.

In the U.S. and Europe, HIV has become a treatable disease, while in the developing world, death is very common, even epidemic, because drugs used to treat HIV are expensive and hard to obtain. Reverse transcriptase inhibitors, such as AZT, ddI, and nevirapine, and protease inhibitors such as indinavir and nelfinavir—both of which act to inhibit the reproduction, and thus spread, of the virus—are the most effective treatments currently available. Antibiotics and other medications are also used to prevent infections. Combinations of these drugs, sometimes called "cocktails," are used to delay the spread of the virus. HIV drugs may cause digestive disorders, headaches, anemia, pancreatic and nerve damage, back pain due to renal colic, elevated blood glucose, and increased cholesterol and triglyceride levels. Herbs may be used to reduce drug side effects and improve quality of life.

Self-Help

- High-potency antioxidant such as Quercenol (use as directed)
- NAC (N-acetylcysteine) (500 to 1,000 mg. per day)

Professional Treatment

- Enhance (3 to 5 tablets four times per day), a clinically studied formula used to improve quality of life
- Clear Heat (2 to 3 tablets four times per day) typically added to Enhance for heat signs

- Polilipid (4 tablets per day) used for increased cholesterol and triglycerides
- Marrow Plus (3 tablets three times per day) for blood deficiency
- Chzyme (2 tablets three times per day) for indigestion
- EPAQ krill oil (3 soft gel capsules per day with meals) to reduce inflammation

Insomnia

According to the American Sleep Disorders Association, more than thirty-five million Americans suffer from chronic insomnia, while another twenty to thirty million suffer shorter-term sleeplessness.[11] Insomnia is simply not getting enough sleep. Typical symptoms include difficulty falling asleep, waking up during the night, and daytime fatigue. Insomnia can be caused by many things, including anxiety, pain, jet lag, change in schedule, habitual napping, drinking excessive amounts of caffeinated beverages, alcohol, medications, sleeping pills, recreational drug use, hormonal disorder, sleep apnea, allergies, and restless leg syndrome. The following suggestions can help promote a more restful sleep.

Some people are night owls, and some are early birds—recognize your leanings, and don't squeeze yourself into a sleep schedule that doesn't suit your natural rhythms. Whatever hours you like to keep, it helps to create a sleep routine and pleasant rituals around going to bed. Try to go to bed and wake up at the same time, regardless of how much, or how little, sleep you have gotten. For example, sleeping in on the weekends is not conducive to a sleep routine.

An ideal routine includes taking a warm bath with calming essential oils such as lavender or lemon balm one hour before bed, followed by a calming tea such as passionflower. A protein shake before bed works for some people, just like the traditional cup of warm milk. It's worth trying for a week to see if it works for you.

If you take natural sleep relaxants, take them before your bath. It is important to take herbs a half hour or more before bed, as they typically take longer than pharmaceuticals to reach effectiveness, so taking them right before bed may be too late.

Some people are very sensitive to light—think about trying blackout curtains, or an eye mask, to keep out ambient light. Use your bed only for sleep and sex, not to watch television, read, or work. Keep work out of the bedroom. Hide distractions such as loud or light-emitting appliances like alarm clocks, computer screens, or clock radios. If you have to have a computer in the bedroom, do something to hide it from view while you're sleeping.

If you do wake up in the night, try to meditate. You will either relax your mind or you will fall asleep—both are highly beneficial. If you don't fall asleep within thirty minutes, get up, go into another room, and read or do some work until you feel tired again. It feels better to get up and get something done than it does to lie in bed, frustrated and tossing and turning.

Don't exercise too late in the day, or too much in general. If you are exercising two hours or more a day, you may need to cut back on exercise to get a decent night's sleep.

Sleeping medications are often habit-forming and addictive, so while they may be useful for short-term use, they are not a long-term solution to sleep problems. People also often use over-the-counter antihistamines to help them sleep, but antihistamines come with a long list of unpleasant side effects, including dry mouth or mucous membranes, headache, vertigo, dizziness, insomnia, jitteriness, drowsiness, nausea, diarrhea, and dyspepsia. Fortunately, there are natural methods that can make sleep easier and more restful.

According to Chinese medicine, insomnia may be caused by fear, or by a lack of nourishment of heart blood or heart yin. In clinical practice, it is common to prescribe multiple herbal formulas for insomnia. For people who have chronic insomnia it may be necessary to use a constitutional formula during the day, and a more sedating formula prior to bed. Chinese herbs typically have fewer side effects than Western pharmaceutical sleep aids, though they also work more slowly. Light boxes (www. northernlighttechnologies.com) can be useful for people with chronic insomnia. They are typically used for thirty minutes when first waking up.

Self-Help

Look for nighttime calcium/magnesium supplements in your health food store or pharmacy, and use with the following supplements.

- Melatonin (.5 to 3 mg.), recommended for short-term use only since melatonin is a hormone. Always start at the lowest dosage.
- Passionflower or lemon balm tea, 1 to 2 cups, one hour before bed
- Valerian (use as directed)
- Kava (use as directed)

Professional Treatment

- Griffonex–5HTP (2 to 3 capsules one hour before bed, and when you wake up during the night)

- Schizandra Dreams (2 to 3 capsules one hour before bed, and when you wake up during the night)

One of the above formulas can be combined with one of the daily tonics below:

- Shen Gem *(gui pi tang)* (3 to 5 tablets three times per day) is a constitutional formula. Treatment used during the day if fatigue, pallor, and difficulty falling asleep.
- Calm Spirit (3 tablets three times per day) is used with yin deficiency characterized by feeling hot at night and waking up frequently.

Kidney Failure

The kidneys filter wastes such as urea, uric acid, and creatine out of the blood, so they can be excreted in the urine. At the same time, the kidneys keep the substances your body needs—sugar, amino acids, calcium, salts—and sends them back to the bloodstream. When the kidneys fail, dangerous levels of wastes and fluids build up in the body.

Diabetes is the most common cause of chronic kidney failure in the U.S. Kidney failure may also be caused by kidney diseases, kidney stones, infection, injury, toxins and medications, high blood pressure, sickle-cell disease, and lupus erythematosus. Other factors that increase risk include excessive use of alcohol, long-term use of pain medications including aspirin, acetaminophen (Tylenol), ibuprofen (Advil, Motrin), and the antibiotics streptomycin or gentamicin.

Acute kidney failure happens suddenly, often after trauma or surgery causing shock or severe bleeding. Chronic kidney failure, on the other hand, happens gradually, over years, and causes no symptoms in the early stages. In chronic kidney failure, symptoms may not show up until the kidney is functioning at 25 percent of normal capacity. About twenty million Americans have chronic kidney failure, and another twenty million are at risk of developing it. Symptoms of chronic kidney failure include high blood pressure, unexplained weight loss, anemia, nausea and vomiting, malaise or fatigue, headaches, decreased urine output, decreased mental sharpness, muscle twitches and cramps, intestinal tract bleeding, yellowish-brown cast to the skin, persistent itching, and sleep disorders. Complications of chronic kidney failure include fluid retention, including congestive heart failure and fluid in the lungs, a sudden rise in blood potassium levels, which can affect heart function, weak bones, stomach ulcers, and nervous system damage.

To diagnose kidney failure, a doctor will order blood and urine tests to check for increased levels of urea and creatine. If those are positive, some kind of imaging might be done, such as ultrasound, CT scan, or MRI, and perhaps a biopsy. Treatment focuses on controlling symptoms and complications and slowing the progression of the disease. First priority is controlling the condition that caused the kidney failure—for example, diabetes or high blood pressure. Decreasing the amount of protein in your diet can slow disease progression and alleviate nausea, vomiting, and low appetite.

End-stage renal disease is diagnosed when blood tests show consistently high levels of urea and creatine. At this point, the kidneys have basically shut down, functioning at less than 10 percent of capacity, and dialysis or a kidney transplant is necessary.

Professional Treatment

◆ L-Carnitine (2 to 10 g. per day) can be used to protect the heart for dialysis patients

- Rehmannia 8 (3 tablets three times per day) is an adjunct formula used to support kidney function. It is typically combined with Cordyceps PS
- Cordyceps PS (2 tablets two times per day) to support kidney function
- Co-Q10 200 mg. per day to improve kidney function

Labyrinthitis

Labyrinthitis is an infection of the looping canals of the inner ear, known collectively as the labyrinth, which controls balance and hearing. Labyrinthitis produces dizziness and extreme difficulties in maintaining balance, nausea, vomiting, hearing loss, and involuntary eye movements. Labyrinthitis is typically caused by bacteria, or occurs secondary to viral meningitis. Standard treatments include rest, anti-nausea drugs, and antibiotics if a bacterial infection is involved.

Professional Treatment

- Flavonex (3 tablets three times per day) to improve circulation to the inner ear
- Clear Phlegm (1 to 2 tablets three to four times per day) especially used if mucus or heavy tongue coating is experienced
- Six Gentlemen is used to prevent fluid build up and supports immune function

Laryngitis

Laryngitis is an infection or irritation of the larynx, which is also known as the "voice box." Laryngitis produces tickling, rawness, and hoarseness of the throat, and a need to clear your throat. Laryngitis can be caused by a cold, flu, bronchitis, pneumonia, excessive talking or singing, allergy, breathing chemicals that irritate the throat, alcohol, smoking, or stomach acid reflux. Laryngitis that is accompanied by a cold or flu usually lasts only a few days. If it lasts longer, see a health professional because antibiotics may be necessary.

Self-Help

- Slippery elm (1 tsp. in boiling water three times per day)
- Echinacea, goldenseal (use as directed)
- Gargle with goldenseal (20 drops in water) several times per day

Professional Treatment

- Cold Away (3 tablets four to six times per day) treats sore throat
- Tremella & American Ginseng (3 to 5 tablets four times per day) for dry cough
- Isatis Gold (3 tablets every two to four hours) treats sore throat and reduces bacterial and viral infections

Leukemia

Leukemia is a cancer of the bone marrow stem cells that make white blood cells. Cancerous stem cells crowd out the stem cells that make red blood cells and platelets, causing anemia and bleeding, while also making too many white blood cells, which cause swelling of the liver and spleen. Leukemia is classified by the stem cells involved, whether lymphocytic (referring to white blood cells) or myelogenous/myeloid (these words both refer to bone marrow, and are used interchangeably), and by the severity of the illness, whether acute or chronic.

Acute leukemia is treated with chemotherapy, because the drugs have a much stronger effect on the cancer cells than the normal cells. However, chemotherapy isn't so effective with chronic leukemia, because the drugs can be as harmful to healthy cells as to the cancer cells, so chronic cases may be treated with blood transfusions and antibiotics. Drugs used in treating leukemia include hydroxyurea, chlorambucil, and prednisone.

In China, herbs have long been used to reduce leukemia symptoms and the side effects of chemotherapy, to support the immune system, and to inhibit the leukemia cells. Nutrition and herbs can relieve symptoms and prolong life span.

In **acute lymphocytic leukemia (ALL),** cells that normally develop into lymphocytes become cancerous, and replace normal cells in the bone marrow. Symptoms may include fatigue, shortness of breath, infection, fever, bleeding, headaches, vomiting, irritability, and joint and bone pain. Laboratory tests and a bone marrow biopsy are the usual methods of diagnosis. The main treatment is chemotherapy, although methotrexate and bone marrow transplants may also be used.

Acute myeloid leukemia (AML) involves myelocytes—cells that usually become bacteria-fighting granulocytes—turning cancerous and replacing normal cells in the bone marrow.

AML may be caused by radiation and chemotherapy. Early symptoms include fatigue, shortness of breath, infection, fever, and bleeding. In addition, there may be headaches, vomiting, and bone and joint pain. Diagnosis is made on the basis of blood tests and bone marrow biopsy. Biomedical treatments involve chemotherapy, blood transfusions, bone marrow transplants, and antibiotics to treat infections.

Chronic lymphocytic leukemia (CLL) is characterized by a high quantity of cancerous lymphocytes and enlarged lymph nodes. The main symptoms are enlarged lymph nodes, fatigue, weight loss, abdominal fullness (caused by an enlarged spleen), skin rashes, and bruising easily. Blood tests and bone marrow biopsy may be performed. CLL usually progresses slowly, but people with CLL are more likely to develop other cancers as well. Treatment depends on the stage and severity of the disease, as people diagnosed with CLL often survive twenty years after the diagnosis is made. Treatment may include using erythropoietin injections or blood transfusions to increase the number of red blood cells; platelet transfusions to increase the number of platelets; and radiation to reduce swelling in the lymph nodes, liver, or spleen. Prednisone or other corticosteroids may be used to reduce the number of lymphocytes. Other treatments may include alkylating agents, alpha interferon, and pentostatin. Infections are treated with antibiotics.

In **chronic myelocytic leukemia (CML),** which progresses faster than CLL, cancerous bone marrow cells produce a large number of abnormal granulocytes. Over time, people with CML may experience fatigue, weight loss, night sweats, loss of appetite, and fullness caused by an enlarged spleen. Pallor, bruising, and bleeding occur when there aren't enough red blood cells and platelets, crowded out by the quickly reproducing granulocytes. If you have CML and experience fever, swollen lymph nodes, or skin nodules filled with leukemic granulocytes, contact your doctor immediately. CML is diagnosed with blood tests, and commonly treated with chemotherapy, radiation, and bone marrow transplant.

Professional Treatment

- Clear Heat for enlarged lymph nodes and heat symptoms (3 tablets three times per day)
- Marrow Plus (3 tablets three times per day) is used in the event of bone marrow suppression or anemia
- Power Mushrooms (2 to 3 tablets three times per day)
- Coriolus PS (3 tablets three times per day) for immune system support
- Ecliptex (2 to 3 tablets three times per day) to reduce liver toxicity
- See protocols in "Cancer" section of this chapter

Case Study

Mary is a forty-one-year-old female whose chief complaints were high liver counts following her first round of chemotherapy to treat leukemia. Her ALT was 375, and her AST was 331; these were both significantly higher than normal; the doctor told her she would not be able to resume chemo until her liver counts reduced. Mary's chemo protocol was cyclophosphamide, daunorubicin, vincristine, prednisone, and L-asparaginase. Her main symptoms were dryness of the throat and sinuses, fatigue, and irritability. Her tongue was red and dry and swollen around the edges; her pulse was choppy.

I recommended Ecliptex (3 tablets four times per day) with Milk Thistle 80 (1 tablet four times per day). Ecliptex is a blend of herbs with proven liver regeneration and repair effects, and Milk Thistle 80 contains 80 percent silymarin, which is also useful in regenerating the liver. After one month of taking the herbs, Mary's liver counts were reduced to 220 and 261, respectively; thus, they had decreased, although they were still above normal. She had greater energy and less dryness, her tongue was less swollen around the edges but otherwise unchanged, and her pulse was still choppy. Mary remained on the herbs for another month and at this point the liver counts had dropped further to 100 and 112, respectively; thus, her chemotherapy treatments were started again. Mary stayed on the herbs for almost a year and was able to normalize her liver counts; in addition, she felt less fatigue and irritability.

Lupus

Lupus is an autoimmune disease that produces chronic inflammation. It affects one to two million Americans, 75 percent of whom are women with a typical age of onset at fifteen to thirty-five. It is hypothesized that lupus may be caused by an unidentified virus, but genetics, hormonal factors, stress, and nutrient deficiencies may also play a role. "It is clear that in social groups where stress is high and antioxidant intake is low, the expression of lupus is greater and the intensity of the syndrome is also stronger," according to Russell M. Jaffe, M.D., Ph.D., president and lab director of Serammune Physicians Lab.[12]

Lupus is characterized by inflammation of the skin, blood vessels, tissues, and joints. Symptoms may include joint pain, muscle weakness, headache, fatigue, poor concentration, hair loss, fever, anemia, chest pain, sores in the mouth, nose, or vagina, and rashes. The name lupus, which is Latin for wolf, originated because the classic butterfly-shaped facial rash gave sufferers a wolf-like appearance. There are two types of lupus: systemic lupus erythematosus (SLE), which affects different parts of the body, and discoid lupus erythematosus (DLE), which affects the skin.

Flare-ups may be triggered by stress, fatigue, infections, chemicals, drug reactions, sun exposure, pregnancy, and childbirth. If you must go out in the sun, wear a sunscreen containing PABA with an SPF of at least 15, wear a hat and sunglasses, and cover your arms and legs. Try to get plenty of sleep to allow your body to recover from daily activities and stress. Tiredness and stress wear down the immune system, which can lead to flare-ups.

Physicians prescribe steroids, immune suppressants, and the anti-malarial drug chloroquine. Both immune suppressants and steroids have significant long-term side effects. Stress reduction and appropriate exercise can reduce flare-ups.

Self-Help

- Omega-3 EPA/DHA fatty acids for anti-inflammatory effects (3 to 10 g. per day of fish oil) or EPAQ krill oil (3 soft gel capsules per day with meals)
- High-potency antioxidant formula such as Quercenol (use as directed)
- Vitamin E (400 to 800 IU daily) is an antioxidant that softens skin and reduces inflammation
- Vitamin B_{12} levels have been found to be low in lupus patients, and B_{12} also treats pernicious anemia (1,000 to 3,000 mcg. daily, sublingual form)

Professional Treatment

- DHEA (25 to 200 mg. per day) is an adrenal hormone that has been found, in double-blind studies, to result in significantly fewer flare-ups for lupus patients than a placebo (sugar pill). Make sure to take DHEA under the care of a holistic physician, because it can cause side effects such as acne, lowered HDL (the good cholesterol), and hormonal irregularities
- EPAQ krill oil (3 soft gel capsules per day with meals)
- Power Mushrooms for autoimmune disease and to improve energy level (3 tablets three times per day)
- Great Yin for yin deficient with dryness and heat signs including rash (3 tablets three times per day)
- Clear Heat used as an adjunct if heat signs (2 to 3 tablets three to four times per day)
- Nine Flavor Tea with dryness (3 tablets three times per day)
- Astra Isatis for immune support (3 tablets three times per day), lymphatic congestion and to improve energy level

Lyme Disease

Lyme disease was named after Lyme, Connecticut, where a cluster of children with arthritis was observed in the 1970s. Lyme disease is transmitted by a tick bite, and is common on the East and West coasts, and in Wisconsin and Minnesota. Lyme disease affects the skin in its early stage, and spreads to the joints and nervous system as it progresses.

The signature symptom of early Lyme disease is a rash that radiates from a tick bite. The rash may be solid red, or look like a bull's-eye, with a red center and outer ring of red. The rash appears one to two weeks after the bite, averages five to six inches in diameter, and persists for about three to five weeks. It may or may not be warm to the touch, but is usually not painful or itchy. Along with the rash, the infected individual may have symptoms including joint and muscle pains, headache, chills, fever, and fatigue, though these symptoms may be mild and easy to overlook.

As the disease progresses, symptoms may include migrating pains in joints and tendons, a stiff, aching neck, tingling or numbness in the extremities, or facial paralysis. The most severe symptoms of Lyme disease may occur weeks or months after the tick bite. These can include severe headaches, painful arthritis and swelling of joints, cardiac abnormalities, and disabling neurological disorders causing confusion, dizziness, memory loss, and mental fog.

Lyme disease resembles many other conditions, and so diagnosis can be difficult. It is sometimes diagnosed on the basis of a blood test, but these tests are not always conclusive. If caught early, antibiotics such as doxycycline or amoxicillin are generally effective. Lyme disease can become debilitating if not caught early, or if the infected individual's immune system is weak. Doctors may treat more severe Lyme disease, with neurological symptoms, with intravenous ceftriaxone or penicillin for four weeks or more. Some patients have symptoms that linger for months or even years following treatment.

Self-Help

◆ To avoid picking up ticks, be careful when walking in wooded areas. Wear long pants tucked into socks, long-sleeve shirts, and shoes. Check yourself and your pets for ticks often.

◆ If you find a tick, remove it immediately with tweezers. If you can't remove it completely, visit a hospital immediately. If fever or other symptoms develop, see a health professional as soon as possible.

Professional Treatment

◆ Power Mushrooms (1 to 3 tablets three times per day) to promote energy
◆ Aquilaria 22 (1 to 3 tablets three times per day) to eliminate toxins and treat constipation
◆ Colostroplex (1 to 4 tablets per day for one year or longer) has been used to improve immune functioning and to eliminate bacteria, viruses, and fungus
◆ CordySeng (1 to 3 tablets two to three times per day) helps replenish energy levels and may protect the heart
◆ Vinpurazine (1 to 4 tablets daily) to improve mental functioning
◆ Ecliptex (1 to 3 tablets three times per day) reduces liver toxicity
◆ AC-Q (2 to 3 tablets three times per day) for joint and muscle pain

Ménière's Disease

Ménière's disease was named after the French physician who first described it in 1861. Its symptoms are related to change in fluid volume in the inner ear "labyrinth," which is responsible for hearing and balance. Symptoms of Ménière's disease include periodic rotatory vertigo or dizziness, fluctuating and progressive low-frequency hearing loss, usually affecting only one ear, tinnitus (ringing in the ears), and a sensation of fullness or pressure in the ear. It most commonly affects people in their forties and fifties, men and women equally. The vertigo can severely disrupt the patient's life, sometimes confining them to bed. Anxiety and depression often accompany severe symptoms.

Ménière's disease is diagnosed with hearing and balance tests. MRIs are used to eliminate a tumor as the cause of the symptoms. Ménière's is treated by reducing fluid retention by cutting consumption of salt, caffeine, and alcohol, with medications to control allergies and improve blood circulation in the inner ear, and by reducing stress. Surgery and injections of the antibiotic gentamicin directly into the middle ear have recently gained popularity as a treatment.

Professional Treatment

- ◆ Drain Dampness (3 tablets three times per day) to reduce fluid retention
- ◆ Formula V (1 to 2 tablets three times per day) to increase blood flow and reduce edema
- ◆ Clear Phlegm (3 tablets three times per day) as an adjunct with mucus and coated tongue
- ◆ Flavonex (2 to 3 tablets three times per day) for circulation

Mononucleosis

Mononucleosis—or mono as it is popularly called—is an infection of the Epstein-Barr virus. The main symptoms are fever, sore throat, fatigue, muscle pain, swollen lymph nodes, nausea, and loss of appetite. There can also be an enlarged spleen, jaundice, headache, cough, and rapid heartbeat. Seek a physician if you have sudden sharp pain in the left upper abdomen, which could signal significant damage to the spleen.

Although mono can affect anyone, teenagers are especially prone. Although many of the symptoms may disappear in ten days, fatigue and weakness may last up to three months. If you or a loved one is suspected to have mono, see a health professional because mono may mimic other infections, including hepatitis and HIV disease. There is currently no medical treatment, though physicians typically recommend rest and plenty of fluids.

Self-Help

♦ Quercenol or broad-spectrum antioxidant formula
♦ Shiitake tea—1 to 3 buttons, simmer in water for 15 minutes, drink broth

Professional Treatment

♦ Astra Isatis (3 tablets three to four times per day) is often an excellent base formula with immune and anti-viral herbs. If heat signs are present, add Clear Heat (2 to 3 tablets three to four times per day)
♦ If cold signs are present, add Power Mushrooms (2 tablets three to four times per day)
♦ Thymus supplements (use as directed)

Multiple Sclerosis (MS)

MS affects an estimated 500,000 Americans, is twice as common in women as in men, and is found more frequently in people of Northern European descent. MS is an autoimmune disease in which immune cells attack the myelin sheaths that insulate nerve cells in the brain and spinal cord, causing inflammation and scarring (sclerosis). The scar tissue slows or blocks the normal transmission of nerve signals. Symptoms vary, depending on the location of the scarring, and may include numbness or weakness of one or more limbs, fatigue, dizziness, tingling or electric-shock sensations, muscle twitches, and impaired vision. As the disease progresses, there may be paralysis, problems with bladder, bowel, and sexual function, slurred speech, and mental changes like memory loss and confusion.

Although the cause has not been determined, there seems to be a predisposition for MS for people with close relatives who have MS. Even then, the disease may lie dormant unless triggered by stress, infections, or exposure to high temperatures.

Anti-Inflammatory Diet

- Eat fresh fish several times per week
- Take fish oil supplements daily such as EPAQ krill oil or cod-liver oil
- Maximize fruits and vegetables
- Limit alcohol, sweets, fruit juices, and fried foods
- Use healthy oils such as olive oil for cooking and flax and sesame oil as a garnish

Holistic researchers believe MS may result from genetics combined with any of the following factors: mercury or other heavy-metal toxicity, low antioxidant status, vitamin D deficiency, exposure to allergens, and exposure to viruses such as chlamydia, pneumonia, herpes, and mycoplasma infection. Food allergies and nutritional deficiencies may also play a role.

MS is difficult to diagnose because its symptoms come and

go, and may even disappear for years at a time. Also, a number of conditions cause symptoms similar to MS, including brain infections found in Lyme disease, AIDS, syphilis, structural abnormalities of the skull or spine, tumors, strokes, ALS (Lou Gehrig's disease), lupus, and arthritis. Physicians evaluate the nervous system and conduct tests such as MRIs and spinal taps to arrive at a diagnosis.

Injections of beta interferons, such as Avonex, Betaseron, and Rebif, can help reduce relapses, but cause flu-like side effects. Daily glatiramer (Copaxone) injections are used as an alternative to beta interferon, with side effects including flushing and shortness of breath after injections. Corticosteroids can reduce inflammation and shorten flare-ups, but long-time steroid use can cause osteoporosis, high blood pressure, increased infections, diabetes, weight gain, fatigue, and ulcers. Muscle relaxants like tizanidine (Zanaflex) and baclofen (Lioresal) help with painful muscle spasms, though tizanidine causes drowsiness and dry mouth, and baclofen often increases weakness in the legs. Fatigue is commonly treated with the antidepressant fluoxetine (Prozac), the anti-viral amantadine (Symmetrel), or the narcolepsy medication modafinil (Provigil), all of which have stimulant properties.

Self-Help

- DHA may protect the brain from heavy metals
- Vitamin D can reduce bone loss—follow instructions on label, and try to get additional vitamin D by spending 15 to 30 minutes in the sun a day
- High-potency antioxidant such as Quercenol (use as directed)
- Vitamin B_{12} sublingual or injection (1,000 to 3,000 mcg. per day)
- Power Mushrooms (1 to 3 tablets three times per day)

Professional Treatment

- Power Mushrooms (1 to 3 tablets three times per day) for autoimmune and energy levels
- EPAQ krill oil (3 soft gel capsules per day with meals) to reduce inflammation
- Mobility 2 (3 tablets three times per day) has anti-inflammatory effects
- Collagenex (2 tablets two times per day) to maintain integrity of cartilage
- Bee sting therapy see American Apitherapy Society

Case Study

Roxanne was diagnosed with multiple sclerosis (MS) thirty years ago. Currently her main symptoms were pain affecting the entire body, fatigue, depression, and lack of appetite. Her tongue was pale and wet; her pulse was slow and slippery. We recommended Power Mushrooms (3 tablets three times per day) for the first week, in order to strongly tonify her immune system and to help her feel less fatigue. We also suggested that Roxanne use 1 Tbsp. per day of cod-liver oil to reduce inflammation. After one week, the fatigue was slightly improved although other symptoms were unchanged. We recommended adding Mobility 2 (2 tablets three times per day) to reduce inflammation and to circulate blood. She remained on the Power Mushrooms and cod-liver oil.

Roxanne came to our clinic on a monthly basis after the first few visits. There was a gradual improvement in most of her symptoms, especially her fatigue.

Myasthenia Gravis

Myasthenia gravis is a chronic autoimmune disease in which antibodies block the receptors for acetylcholine, which activates muscle contraction at the junction where nerve cells connect with the muscles they control. Although it may affect any voluntary muscle, myasthenia gravis commonly causes weakness in muscles that control eyes and eyelids, facial expressions, and swallowing. Myasthenia gravis most commonly affects women under forty and men over sixty, though it can occur at any age. Because weakness is a symptom common to many disorders, diagnosis can take a couple of years. Physicians should suspect myasthenia gravis when symptoms include eye problems, and weakness without any change in the patient's ability to feel textures. Doctors may order blood tests for acetylcholine receptor antibodies; the edrophonium test for a chemical that temporarily relieves weakness in patients with myasthenia gravis; single-fiber electromyography (EMG); and CT or MRI scans of the thymus to check for a growth or abnormality.

Myasthenia gravis can be controlled with anticholinesterase agents such as neostigmine and pyridostigmine to improve neuromuscular transmission, or immunosuppressive drugs such as prednisone, cyclosporine, and azathioprine to suppress the abnormal antibodies. The thymus gland show signs of abnormal immune activity in people with myasthenia gravis, and in fact, removing the thymus improves symptoms in 50 percent of patients. Other treatments include plasmapheresis and high-dose immunoglobulin therapy.

Professional Treatment

- EPAQ krill oil (3 soft gel capsules per day with meals) to reduce inflammation
- Power Mushrooms for autoimmune diseases, promotes energy levels
- Cogni-Spark (1 to 2 capsules two times per day) to maintain cognitive functions, may improve neuromuscular transmission

Neuropathy/Nerve Pain

Peripheral neuropathy refers to a problem with the peripheral sensory, motor, and autonomic nerves, which run from the brain and spinal cord throughout the body. Symptoms of peripheral neuropathy include tingling and numbness in the hands and feet, pain that may be burning, shooting, throbbing, or aching, sensitivity to touch, muscle weakness, twitching, or cramping.

Neuropathy can be caused by a long list of disorders, with diabetes at the top of that list. Neuropathy can result from a variety of viral infections, including shingles, Epstein-Barr virus, and cytomegalovirus, all of which can damage nerves and cause sharp pain. HIV can cause several different patterns of neuropathy, each identified with a specific stage of immunodeficiency disease. Additionally, neuropathy commonly occurs as a side effect of HIV drugs, and of chemotherapy drugs used to treat cancer. Lyme disease is a bacterial infection known to cause painful neuropathy, often within a few weeks of the infectious tick bite. Viral and bacterial infections may also provoke autoimmune disorders, causing the immune system to attack the nerves. The acute inflammation associated with Guillain-Barré syndrome can also damage peripheral nerve fibers.

Pain due to neuropathy is difficult to control, and can undermine emotional well-being. Neuropathic pain is often worse at night, so it often disrupts sleep as well. If the pain is mild, over-the-counter analgesics may help. More severe pain may be addressed with mexiletine (though it can have severe side effects); anti-epileptic drugs such as gabapentin (Neurontin), phenytoin, and carbamazepine; and the tricyclic antidepressant amitriptyline.

Self-Help

♦ Vitamin B complex (use as directed) B12 (1,000 to 3,000 mcg. per day), and folate (folic acid) (800 mcg. per day) may help alleviate neuropathy symptoms. Supplements shown to have some effect on neuropathy include magnesium (200 to 800 mg. per day), alpha-lipoic acid (300 to 900 mg. per day), and gamma linolenic acid (use as directed)

Professional Treatment

♦ Channel Flow (2 to 3 tablets three to four times per day) if sharp, stabbing pain
♦ Clear Heat (2 to 3 tablets three to four times per day) if heat signs
♦ Marrow Plus (2 to 3 tablets three to four times per day) if blood deficiency
♦ EPAQ krill oil (3 soft gel capsules per day with meals) has anti-inflammatory effects and can be used with the above-mentioned protocols

Parasites

Parasites are a growing problem in developed countries due to an increase in air travel and to water supplies infected by animal waste. Secondary factors are inadequate sterilization and poor hygiene practices at restaurants and day care centers, and drinking untreated water while hiking or camping. Common symptoms are digestive complaints that don't clear up, headache, fatigue, muscle aches, joint pain, and food and environmental sensitivities and allergies. If you have had a chronic digestive condition that has resisted treatment, and have traveled to Asia, South America, or Africa, it is very likely you have a parasitic condition. The same is true if you've consumed untreated water while camping or hiking.

Unfortunately, many physicians in the U.S. are not aware of the rising incidence of parasite infections. Even as far back as 1976, the Centers for Disease Control (CDC) reported that one of every six people tested in the U.S. at random had one or more parasites. One type of infection, giardiasis, is so common in some areas that almost the entire indigenous population host this microorganism. Also known as "Montezuma's Revenge" or the "Delhi Belly," giardiasis can cause violent cramping and diarrhea that continues despite the use of over-the-counter remedies. Giardia organisms can be found in mountain streams, and more alarming is the fact that they can infect city water systems, since giardia is not killed by chlorination. In day care centers giardia and other parasites may be spread by direct contact with feces during diaper changing, as well as by children coming in contact with feces and then putting their hands in their mouths, touching toys or drinking faucets, and engaging in other shared contact.

The immune-compromised are especially vulnerable to parasitic infections, including two in particular—toxoplasmosis, which is transmitted by cats, and cryptosporidiosis, which is acquired through drinking water. Parasites can also be passed through sexual contact. Improper cooking and preparation of foods is another possible source of parasitic transmission. If you enjoy sushi, you should always eat at a reputable restaurant where the chefs practice proper food preparation and sanitary habits, such as frequent hand washing.

Parasites can wreak havoc in the body. Some parasitic infections can be fatal if untreated. Parasites can destroy cells and produce toxic substances. They irritate the body's tissues, causing inflammatory reactions. Untreated infections result in the body's immune system producing too many specialized white blood cells, called eosinophils. Eosinophils can cause tissue damage as they multiply to wipe out the parasites, resulting in pain and inflammation. Also, the immune system becomes exhausted in its intense effort to battle parasitic infection.

Flagyl (metronidazole) is the most common drug used in the U.S. to treat parasites, but it has many side effects. Also, many parasites are Flagyl resistant. What can you do if you have unrelieved digestive disorders or other strange symptoms that have remained untreatable, especially if you have been exposed to one of the above infection pathways? Find a holistic practitioner who can adequately diagnose parasites, or go to a university-affiliated hospital or clinic that has a department of parasitology or tropical medicine.

Preventing Parasites

◆ Filter water. This is especially necessary for the immune-compromised and international travelers. Bottled water may not be pure, or bottles may not be properly sterilized. Take along a water sterilization kit (camping stores often

provide information about which kits and filters are appro-
priate for your needs)
- Be careful about eating out. Eat only properly cooked
foods when you are unsure of the cleanliness standards
- Peel vegetables and fruits
- Make sure you have separate cutting surfaces for meats and
vegetables. These areas should be pet-free
- Have household employees tested for parasites
- Have pets checked on a regular basis for parasites
- Keep pets away from food preparation areas
- Never kiss pets or allow them to sleep with your family
- Protect children from animal droppings
- Immune-compromised persons should not handle cat litter.
If this is not possible, use surgical gloves and wear a face
mask, while keeping the litter as far away from the body as
possible. Wash hands thoroughly afterward
- Practice safe sex

Symptoms and Treatments

- Chlorine food bath: Use 1 to 2 tsp. of bleach to one gallon
of water. Leafy vegetables, thin-skinned fruits, and all
meats (separate baths for different meats) should be placed
in the bath for twenty minutes. Then place in clear water
for ten minutes. Thoroughly clean and dry all food treated
this way. This procedure can be used by susceptible
individuals, and those living in areas of known infestation.
- Freezing: Freeze fish for forty-eight hours, beef and pork
for twenty-four hours. This procedure will kill any larvae.
- Cooking: Make sure meat is thoroughly cooked (no pink
showing). When eating out, request that meat be cooked
well done. At home, cook meat at a minimum of 325°F

(161°C), fish at 400°F (202°C). Beef, lamb, veal, and pork should be cooked to an internal temperature of 170°F (76°C).

Professional Treatment

- Aquilaria 22 (1 to 3 tablets three times per day) plus Artestatin (start at 1 tablet per day, increase to 6 to 9 per day over a two-week period) can be taken before meals
- With constipation, increase Aquilaria 22, decrease Artestatin dosages
- With diarrhea, increase Artestatin, decrease Aquilaria 22 dosages
- Use Quiet Digestion (2 tablets three times per day or as needed) for cramping, intestinal gas, and poor digestion
- Use Colostroplex (1 to 6 tablets per day) to help bind and eliminate toxins. Decrease dosage if constipation results
- After three months of Artestatin and Aquilaria 22, if parasites are still evident, consider Biocidin (use as directed) or black walnut hulls (start at 1 capsule, try to increase to 10 capsules daily). I recommend these products be taken consecutively, not at the same time. Always begin anti-parasitic herbs at a reduced dosage to avoid unpleasant reactions
- As an adjunct, 2 cloves of raw chopped or chewed garlic (not heated) can be taken. Garlic is considered effective for amebic dysentery and other parasite infections. Note that prepared garlic formulas may not be effective for parasites, and some individuals are sensitive to garlic
- EPAQ krill oil and other fish oil products may be used as an adjunct, as there is experimental evidence that fish oil helps to eliminate parasites

Case Studies

Case #1

Doug, fifty, suffered intense lower right quadrant pain and high fever once or twice a year, lasting four to seven days. These attacks began following a trip to China several years ago. Conventional medical tests were negative for ulcers, parasites, and appendicitis. A chiropractor told him that he had a fungal infection of the ileo-cecal valve. Doug had a history of hepatitis, although his liver enzymes were not elevated. He had tried various herbal combinations for the pain, but the condition persisted. Traditional Chinese diagnosis found that his pulse was wiry and his tongue flabby (revealing dampness) and red around the edges, with a greasy coating. I prescribed a general cleansing protocol that addressed both parasites and candida, surmising that he had contracted a parasitic infection in China that was undiagnosable by Western tests. As the primary remedy, I recommended Aquilaria 22 (2 tablets three times per day), since his stools were normal, to be taken for three months. He was also given Artestatin (1 tablet three times per day) for two months, followed by Phellostatin (2 tablets three times per day) for one month. After two weeks, he reported some cramping, which he believed was due to the herbal formulas. I suggested that he reduce the dosage of Artestatin to 2 tablets a day, and if he still experienced cramping to reduce the dosage further (Artestatin is especially effective in killing amoebic cysts; however, cramping is a sign that the dosage should be reduced). I indicated that he could also reduce the dosage of Aquilaria 22. Since I believed that he might have been having a die-off reaction, I started him on the preparation Ecliptex (2 tablets three times per day), which is useful for detoxifying the liver.

Two weeks later he developed a cold of the wind-cold variety, so I recommended Isatis Gold (3 tablets four to six times per day), and told him to temporarily discontinue the anti-parasitic herbs. As he was having loose stools, fatigue, and abdominal pain following the initial cold symptoms, I recommended Quiet Digestion and Ease 2 (2 tablets three times per day of each formula); the latter is a traditional remedy used to address lingering cold symptoms. He reported feeling better a few days later after using this protocol. He felt less achy, but still experienced some loose stools, so he continued on the formulas for a few more days. When he felt better, I advised him to resume the Aquilaria 22 (1 tablet three times per day) and Quiet Digestion (2 tablets three times per day) for a week before going back to the Artestatin. He continued to take the three remedies for a few more weeks. As he was about to go on a business trip and had no digestive symptoms, I recommended he continue to take the Aquilaria 22 (1 tablet three times per day), Artestatin (1 tablet per day), Ecliptex (2 tablets three times per day), and Quiet Digestion (as needed). When he returned from his business trip, he reported that the Quiet Digestion had given him symptomatic relief on a few occasions. He asked my opinion about addressing the fungal infection and I indicated that Aquilaria 22 and Phellostatin had anti-fungal properties. His new regimen therefore was Aquilaria 22 (1 tablet three times per day), Phellostatin (1 tablet three times per day), Ecliptex (2 tablets three times per day), and Quiet Digestion (as needed).

A few weeks later, Doug contracted food poisoning. I told him to take Quiet Digestion (2 tablets four to six times per day), and to chew 1 tablet of Aquilaria 22 every few hours. He reported great relief. He remained on a maintenance protocol of Aquilaria 22 (1 tablet three times per day), Phellostatin (1 tablet three times per day), and Ecliptex (2 tablets three times per day) for another month. As of this writing, he has not had an episode of appendicitis-like pain in one year. He uses Quiet Digestion symptomatically for digestive upset.

Discussion: Doug's case demonstrates that anti-parasitic formulas should be administered long term for best results. Also, those who have parasitic infections are more susceptible to colds, the flu, and food poisoning. Finally, it is not uncommon to have parasitic and fungal infections simultaneously.

Case #2

Samantha, thirty-two years old, is a health professional who developed chronic diarrhea after a vacation to Mexico four years ago. Following a thorough biomedical evaluation, she was treated with Flagyl. However, she continued having up to ten episodes of watery stools per day. She also suffered from fatigue, occasional headaches, and joint pain. Traditional Chinese diagnosis found that her pulse was weak and slow, and her tongue pale and swollen. I recommended a combination of Source Qi formula (3 tablets three times per day for the first week, 5 tablets three times per day thereafter), along with an herbal anti-parasitic, Artestatin (1 tablet three times per day). The first week she reported cramps after taking the herbs, so I suggested reducing the dosage of Artestatin to 1 tablet per day and maintaining the Source Qi dosage (3 tablets three times per day). By the end of the second week, her stools were more formed, but the frequency—especially in the morning—was unchanged. At this point, Colostroplex (1 tablet three times per day) was added to the existing protocol. At the end of the fourth week, the urgency and number of stools had decreased. She was referred to a lab specializing in parasitic diseases, where they found the presence of Histoplasma capsulatum, a fungus. Therefore, I suggested increasing the dosage of Artestatin (2 tablets per day), as well as taking the herbal anti-fungal Biocidin (2 drops on a cracker with meals). She also continued taking Colostroplex (1 tablet three times per day) and Source Qi (3 tablets three times per day).

At the end of the third month, her stools were mostly normal, with an occasional bout of watery stools. The joint pain and headaches had disappeared. She continues to take the herbs until all symptoms are alleviated and parasite tests are negative.

Pneumonia

Pneumonia is an inflammation of lung tissue. There are more than fifty different types of pneumonia, which may be caused by bacteria, viruses, and chemical irritants. Symptoms include cough with bloody sputum, shortness of breath, chest pain, fever, chills, bluish skin (cyanosis), and confusion. Diagnosis is made by listening to your chest, examining the lungs with a bronchoscopy tube, bacterial culture, and blood test. Antibiotics are administered if you are found to have bacteria. Pneumonia can be life-threatening, so it is important that you see a health professional if you think you may have pneumonia, especially for young children, seniors, and anyone with a weak immune system. The following approaches should be used in addition to biomedical approaches.

Self-Help

- NAC (N-acetylcysteine) (500 to 1,000 mg. per day) plus a high-potency antioxidant such as Quercenol (use as directed)

Professional Treatment

- Clear Air (3 tablets four to six times per day) if coughing and chest discomfort
- Cordyceps PS (2 to 3 tablets two to three times per day) has an anti-bacterial effect and improves oxygen utilization; or CordySeng (2 tablets three times per day) to improve oxygen utilization
- EPAQ krill oil (1 to 3 soft gel capsules per day with meals)
- Tremella & American Ginseng (3 to 5 tablets four times per day) for dry cough and feeling hot at night

Case Studies

Case #1

Eva was a sixty-eight-year-old postal worker with a history of upper respiratory infections. Three months before visiting our clinic, she had contracted pneumonia, for the second time that year, and was currently exhibiting signs of flu. She was exhausted, running a fever, and had a headache with sinus pain. Her mucus was yellow, and her skin felt hot and clammy. Eva's pulse was weak and slightly rapid; her tongue was red with a heavy yellow coat. We recommended Isatis Gold (2 tablets four times per day) and Nasal Tabs 2 (2 tablets four times per day). We also suggested she drink three cups a day of peppermint tea. When she returned to our clinic one week later as scheduled, she remarked that she felt better two days after beginning the herbs. Her symptoms were dry barking cough, and feeling hot at night. There was minimal phlegm production except upon awakening. Her pulse was weak, and her tongue was normal colored, dry, with a thin dark yellow coat. We suggested

Tremella & American Ginseng to nourish yin and reduce dryness (3 tablets three times per day) and CordySeng Powder (½ tsp. stirred into hot water three times per day) to strongly tonify her lungs. She returned in two weeks feeling better than she had in a long time. Her dry cough was less frequent and less severe. Her pulse was weak, and her tongue was normal colored, dry, with a slight white coat. We treated Eva for six months, modifying the protocol slightly. During the treatment time, she reported no further infections, and her general vitality had increased noticeably.

Case #2
Rich was a thirty-nine-year-old male who had completed both radiation and chemotherapy for Hodgkin's lymphoma. As a result, his immune system was weakened and he had contracted pneumonia, which required hospitalization. He was currently on oral antibiotics. His symptoms were shortness of breath, exhaustion, productive cough especially in the morning and a dry cough at night, dizziness, and some indigestion. Rich was running a low-grade fever in the afternoon and felt cold on the outside and hot on the inside. His pulse was floating and weak; his tongue was red with geographic coating that appeared gray. We recommended Ease 2 (5 tablets three times per day) to help to harmonize the interior and exterior, with Cordyceps PS (2 tablets three times per day) to improve his breathing, reduce his cough, and tonify his immune system. After one week there was a slight improvement in his exhaustion, breathing, and indigestion. His pulse was sinking, thin, and weak; his tongue was red. At this point we substituted Marrow Plus (3 tablets three times per day), a strong blood-building formula, for Ease 2. Marrow Plus was targeted toward reducing the sensation of cold exterior and warm interior and the dizziness. He maintained on the Cordyceps PS. After one month Rich was feeling better, though still tired. His pulse

267

was slightly stronger, and his tongue was unchanged. He maintained on the herbs for several additional months.

Polymyalgia Rheumatica

Polymyalgia rheumatica is an inflammatory disorder that primarily affects older adults, with the average onset around age seventy. It causes muscle aches and stiffness especially in the hips, thighs, shoulders, upper arms, and neck, which may be accompanied by fatigue, fever, and weight loss. The symptoms often appear suddenly, and can often go away just as suddenly after a year or more. To diagnose polymyalgia rheumatica, doctors may look for an elevated erythrocyte sedimentation rate. They may also test for rheumatoid factor, which is positive in rheumatoid arthritis, but usually negative with polymyalgia rheumatica. To control the symptoms, Western physicians commonly prescribe low doses of the steroid prednisone, and anti-inflammatories such as aspirin and ibuprofen.

Professional Treatment

- Mobility 2 (2 to 4 tablets three times per day) to reduce inflammation, plus Clear Heat (2 to 3 tablets three to four times per day) if heat signs, or Channel Flow (2 tablets three times per day) with debilitating pain
- EPAQ krill oil (1 to 3 soft gel capsules per day with meals) to reduce inflammation
- Collagenex (2 tablets twice per day) to reduce inflammation and joints and surrounding areas

Psoriasis

Psoriasis is characterized by elevated, red, and inflamed patches, which are often accompanied by silvery scales. The patches are usually asymptomatic, except during flare-ups, when itching and a burning sensation may be present. Psoriasis can be found any-where on the body, though typically the knees, elbows, and scalp are affected. Fingernails can show yellowing, with ridges, and pitting of the nail bed. With psoriatic arthritis, there may be joint pain and stiffness. A skin biopsy may be done to confirm a visual diagnosis. Medical attention should be sought immediately if pso-riasis develops over a large portion of the body.

The biomedical cause of psoriasis appears to be an autoim-mune phenomenon. Also, persons with psoriasis often have a family history for the disease. Flare-ups of psoriasis can be trig-gered by emotional stress, skin damage, cold weather, physical illness, or other factors. Medications such as lithium, quinidine, and drugs that treat high blood pressure and inflammation are also known to exacerbate psoriasis.

Biomedical treatment of psoriasis involves topical agents when the affected areas are limited to less than 20 percent of the body surface. Such agents include emollients, keratolytics, corticos-teroids, and coal tar, among others. Systemic and more aggres-sive treatment is used for psoriasis that covers more than 20 percent of the body surface. Such treatment involves phototherapy and medications such as retinoids (acitretin), antimetabolites (methotrexate), and calcineurin inhibitors (cyclosporine). Side effects are often associated with long-term administration of all medications, whether topical or systemic. For example, corti-costeroids often become ineffective and may exacerbate psoria-sis by masking symptoms.

Psoriasis can be a debilitating disease physically and emotion-ally because of the unsightly blemishes. Therefore, complementary therapies such as acupuncture, meditation, and yoga are helpful. An elimination diet may get to the root of the problem, since there is anecdotal evidence that diet and nutrition are causal factors for psoriasis flare-ups (see Chapter Four, "Digestive Clearing Diet").

Self-Help

- Oatmeal baths, to soothe psoriatic areas (follow label directions)
- Black currant oil (3,000 mg. daily)
- Pine tar soap (follow label directions)
- Zinc, antioxidant supplements, and a multi mineral supplement (follow label directions)
- Smilax (sarsaparilla) (½ to 1 tsp. three times a day; reduce dosage if diarrhea occurs)
- Flaxseed oil (1 to 3 Tbsp. daily) taken with vitamin E (400 to 800 IU daily), or EPAQ krill oil (1 to 3 soft gels per day with meals), or fish oil concentrate (3 to 10 g. daily)

Professional Treatment

- Skin Balance (2 to 3 tablets three to four times per day)
- For heat signs, add Clear Heat (1 to 2 tablets three times per day)
- For dryness, add Marrow Plus (2 to 3 tablets four times per day)
- Mobility 2 (3 tablets three to four times per day) for swollen joints
- Zaocys (3 tablets three to four times per day) for psoriatic arthritis

- Tamu Oil (use as directed three times per day) over affected areas
- Resinall K: Apply undiluted directly to affected areas (one to three times daily). If skin is too sensitive to undiluted Resinall K, then dilute 1 part Resinall K with 3 parts safflower or extra virgin olive oil and apply to affected areas (one to three times daily)

Case Studies

Case #1

Steve, a fifty-eight-year-old professional, had psoriasis for more than twenty years. His main symptoms were dry, reddish-purple lesions on his legs, arms, hands, and body. The lesions were itchy whenever they flared up. He was about twenty pounds overweight and drank alcohol regularly. Traditional Chinese medicine diagnosis revealed that his pulse was wiry and irregular, and his tongue was purple.

We suggested that Steve drink more water and stop drinking alcohol. We suggested the digestive clearing program, and that he try limiting his consumption of wheat-containing foods. We also recommended that he incorporate more fatty fish into his diet. He was asked to take Skin Balance (2 tablets three times per day), Mobility 2 (3 tablets three times per day), and a supplement high in EPA and DHA (3 capsules daily with meals) in order to control the inflammatory response.

After three weeks Steve reported that the lesions were less itchy and red. However, he felt agitated from following the digestive clearing program and from not having alcohol for one week. We noticed that he had smoked a cigarette in the parking lot while waiting for his appointment. When we inquired, he said that for several months he had been trying to cut down to a few cigarettes per day, but that not drinking alcohol was increasing his cigarette cravings. His pulse was more wirey, and his tongue was dry and purple. We suggested he continue the herbs at the same dosage, and increase the EPA/DHA to 6 capsules daily with meals. We also referred him to an acupuncturist to help ease the cigarette cravings and to treat the neck pain he was also experiencing.

Steve returned in three weeks showing considerable improvement. The skin lesions were starting to shrink; they were mostly pink instead of reddish-purple, and were less itchy. His pulse was less wiry than at his previous visits, but his tongue was unchanged. The acupuncture treatments helped him cut down to one cigarette a day, and reduced his neck pain. He abandoned the digestive clearing program after two weeks, but noticed a correlation between alcohol and wheat consumption and the itching. Although Steve was willing to eliminate bread from his diet, he did not want to eliminate alcohol entirely. We recommended that he continue on the Skin Balance (2 tablets four times per day), Mobility 2 (3 tablets four times per day), and EPA/DHA (6 capsules per day).

After two more months, all Steve's symptoms were improving, so we adjusted his herbal protocol to Skin Balance (2 tablets four times per day), Mobility 2 was stopped, and Marrow Plus (2 tablets four times per day) was added to build his blood. The EPA/DHA dosage remained the same. He continued taking the herbs for six months with total resolution of the psoriasis.

Discussion: Steve's tongue and lesions were purplish, indicating blood stasis, while his being overweight and the pressure of a lingering condition (the psoriasis) indicated dampness. The formula Skin Balance was used to clear the liver: according to the TCM, alcohol is too warming both to the liver and to the body in general. Although Steve was reluctant to eliminate alcohol totally, he was able to reduce his consumption to one to two drinks on the weekends only. This helped keep the psoriasis under control.

The formula Mobility 2 was used to increase blood circulation and drain dampness, and Marrow Plus was selected to help tonify blood in order to relieve itching. A six-month course of treatment is not unusual for stubborn cases of psoriasis.

Case #2

Edwina, a forty-two-year-old musician, suffered from psoriasis for thirty-seven years. The lesions affected her entire body and were especially severe on her arms and legs, where the plaques were purple, thick, and scaly. During flare-ups, her skin was very itchy, particularly at night. Flare-ups were treated with ultraviolet radiation and the corticosteroid, triamcinolone. She was aware that corn, chocolate, fruit, wheat, and peanuts made her symptoms worse. She also complained of poor digestion and abdominal pain, and occasional hot flashes, as she was perimenopausal. Edwina led a hectic life — teaching during the day, and performing in the evenings, in addition to traveling to performances. Thus, it was no surprise that when she came to our clinic she indicated that for more than a year she had been experiencing fatigue with difficulty rising in the morning. Traditional Chinese medicine diagnosis revealed that her pulse was weak and slow, and her tongue was pink, dry, and cracked, with a yellow coating.

After evaluating her overall situation, in particular her diet, we recommended that Edwina eat more lean meat and salmon, as she was consuming a preponderance of carbohydrates. When she was on the road, she usually ate things that triggered flare-ups of her psoriasis. We also urged her to chew her food carefully, as she was prone to eating quickly. She was also asked to take the formulas Colostroplex (1 tablet per day), Skin Balance (2 tablets three times per day), and Quiet Digestion (1 to 2 tablets

273

three times per day). She was instructed to start with 2 tablets of Skin Balance three times per day, but to reduce to 1 tablet three times per day if she developed loose stools.

After two weeks Edwina reported her skin was much less itchy; however, she complained of stomach pain. Her pulse was wiry, slightly irregular, and weak in the first and third positions. Her tongue was still dry, pink, and cracked, with a slightly yellow coating. We recommended she continue with the herbal protocol. To address the stomach pain, we suggested she not eat so much during her evening meal. Two weeks later, the lesions on her legs had totally disappeared, and she reported that the itching had improved 90 percent. With past flare-ups, this degree of improvement had usually been attained only with triamcinolone and ultraviolet radiation. This time, by adding the herbal protocol, she required only triamcinolone and many fewer UV treatments.

At this point she reported that bleeding hemorrhoids were her principal complaint, something that she had not indicated when she first came to the clinic. Sometimes she had to get up as many as ten times a night with the urge to defecate. Her pulse was still weak and slow, and her tongue was now pale with a dry, gray coating. We urged her to undergo standard biomedical tests to rule out other possible causes of blood in the stool. We also suggested she reduce Skin Balance (to 1 tablet three times per day), increase Colostroplex (to 4 tablets per day), increase Quiet Digestion (1 to 3 tablets three times per day), and add Formula H (3 tablets three times a day), a formula specific for hemorrhoids.

Three weeks later, the psoriasis was totally eliminated. During this time, Edwina had decided to go on a three-day vegetable broth fast, which had greatly helped reduce her hemorrhoid symptoms. But now she was constipated. The medical tests to determine the cause of blood in the stool were inconclusive. Her pulse was now thin, and her tongue was still pale and dry. At this time, Edwina discontinued treatment, as her psoriasis was in remission.

Discussion: As is typical of many persons with psoriasis, Edwina's flare-ups were tied to emotional stress and a poor diet, although in her case, it appeared that her diet was the more significant factor in the flare-ups. As an example, she used chocolate as an instant energy boost, particularly when she was traveling. But she would end up paying for it a few days later by experiencing a flare-up. Once her diet was under control, the skin lesions began healing, and the flare-ups decreased in frequency and severity. Using herbal formulas such as Quiet Digestion helped make the food she was sensitive to more tolerable. Skin Balance was used not only to heal her skin, but to promote regular bowel movements so that toxins were eliminated through the stool instead of the skin.

Reiter's Syndrome

Reiter's syndrome—also called reactive arthritis—is a kind of arthritis that occurs as a reaction to an infection, and may be accompanied by conjunctivitis and urinary tract inflammation. Reiter's syndrome is most commonly triggered by chlamydia trachomatis, and is most common in men between the ages of twenty and forty. It typically causes pain and inflammation in the knees, ankles, and feet, and tendinitis, particularly in the Achilles tendon. Urinary tract inflammation can cause an increased need to urinate, a burning sensation with urination, prostatitis with fever and chills, and discharge from the penis.

Reiter's syndrome is difficult to diagnose, with no specific laboratory test to confirm that a person has it. A doctor will typically order several blood tests to rule out look-alike conditions such as rheumatoid arthritis or lupus. A high erythrocyte

sedimentation rate indicates inflammation in the body, and a doctor may also test for infections associated with Reiter's, such as
chlamydia. X-rays can detect some of the symptoms of Reiter's
syndrome such as inflammation and swelling.

Inflammation symptoms associated with Reiter's syndrome
may be treated with NSAIDs, steroid injections, and topicals.
Prescription NSAIDs that have been effective with Reiter's include
indomethacin and tolmetin. Corticosteroid injections into affected
joints may be used for inflammation that doesn't respond to
NSAIDs. For the small percentage of patients with severe symptoms that don't respond to other treatments, immunosuppressive
medications such as sulfasalazine and methotrexate may help.
Gentle exercise can help strengthen muscles around joints and
improve range of motion.

Self-Help

◆ High-potency antioxidant such as Quercenol (use as
  directed)

Professional Treatment

◆ EPAQ krill oil (3 soft gel capsules per day with meals)
◆ Akebia Moist Heat (3 tablets three times per day) for
  urinary tract infections
◆ Mobility 2 (2 to 4 tablets three times per day) to reduce
  inflammation, plus Clear Heat (2 to 3 tablets three to four
  times per day) if heat signs

Case Study

Rick was a thirty-eight-year-old engineer who was diagnosed with Reiter's syndrome. His main symptoms were joint pain, urethritis, and conjunctivitis although he was not having symptoms, as they were controlled by antibiotics. The reason for his consultation was that he had been on antibiotics for the past four years. The antibiotic he was taking, doxycycline, is contraindicated in sun exposure; therefore, he did not feel he could exercise outdoors, something he enjoyed. Lack of exercise contributed to his weight gain. In addition, he felt that the medication was causing irritable bowel syndrome, his main symptoms being intestinal cramping and diarrhea. Traditional Chinese diagnosis revealed Rick's tongue was red with a yellow coating, and his pulse was slippery. We recommended that he check with his doctor about stopping the antibiotic; he said his doctor agreed that he could stop the antibiotic, but if his symptoms of Reiter's returned he would need to be put back on the antibiotic. We suggested that Rick start reducing the antibiotic by taking it every other day instead of every day. We next recommended that he take the herbal formula Unlocking (4 tablets three times per day), as it is used for chronic urinary pain and also helps rid the body of heat, along with probiotic PB-8 (4 capsules daily). We also recommended Colostroplex (2 tablets two times per day) to help reduce diarrhea and help eliminate bacteria. After two weeks there was little change; however, he felt he was having less intestinal cramping and diarrhea. He maintained on all supplements and herbs. After another two weeks, he said he was ready to stop the doxycycline. We suggested he take the antibiotic every three days. After three weeks, he reported that he had stopped the antibiotic against our suggestion. As he felt normal, he was wondering when he could go off the herbs. His pulse felt normal, and his tongue was unchanged. We suggested that he maintain on the probiotics, and that he reduce the Colostroplex to 2 tablets daily, and Unlocking to 3 tablets two times per day. After two weeks he called to say he was starting to have urethritis symptoms and needed to start back on the antibiotics every day. When we saw him next he was discouraged that the herbs "didn't work." I explained that one of the reasons we wanted him to take the antibiotics every other day and then every third day was we were afraid that his body had gotten dependent on the antibiotics, making it imperative that he reduce them slowly. He said that he'd try better next time.

We treated Rick over nine months; the second time around, he was more compliant at reducing the antibiotics more gradually. After he had been off antibiotics for two weeks, his tongue was normal with a white-yellow coat, and his pulse was slippery. As the heat signs were no longer present, we changed his protocol to Shen Ling (3 tablets three times per day), which tonifies the spleen and rids the body of dampness. He maintained on Colostroplex and probiotics. He had been off antibiotics completely for three months when he developed a sinus infection requiring antibiotics. As he was now using antibiotics acutely and not chronically, we did not think he needed to gradually reduce the dosing of antibiotics. As he was now complaining of dry coughing and sinuses, and his tongue was red with yellow coating and his pulse slippery, we changed his protocol to Lily Bulb (3 tablets three times per day) while he maintained on the Colostroplex and probiotics.

Rheumatoid Arthritis (RA)

Rheumatoid arthritis is an autoimmune disease that causes inflammation of the joints, resulting in pain, stiffness, and swelling, and can eventually deform the surrounding bones. In addition, there may be fatigue, especially in the early afternoon. Rheumatoid arthritis develops in about 1 percent of the population, and is more common in women and individuals twenty-five to fifty years of age.

Rheumatoid arthritis may develop suddenly, or over time. When a joint on one side is affected, the corresponding joint on the other side is also affected. Fingers, toes, hands, feet, wrists, elbows, and ankles typically become inflamed first. Pain is likely to be worst just after waking up in the morning or after periods of inactivity. About one-third of people with RA have nodules under the skin. Low-grade fever and nerve damage or leg ulcers may be present. Some people develop lung and heart problems, swollen lymph nodes, Sjögren's syndrome, or eye inflammation.

Many conditions resemble RA, including other forms of arthritis, Lyme disease, Reiter's syndrome, and rheumatic fever. Laboratory tests and X-rays are standard approaches for making a positive diagnosis. For example, seven out of ten patients are positive for rheumatoid factor, an antibody in the blood. Biomedical approaches include anti–inflammatories, steroids, and immunosuppressive drugs. Other approaches may include gold compounds, hydroxychloroquine, penicillamine, and sulfasalazine. Light exercise, especially swimming, water aerobics, and physical therapy can be very beneficial.

Self-Help

- Fish oil supplements (3 to 10 g. per day) or EPAQ krill oil (3 soft gel capsules per day with meals)
- Anti-inflammatory diet (diet listed under "Multiple Sclerosis")
- High-potency antioxidant such as Quercenol (use as directed)

Professional Treatment

- EPAQ krill oil (3 soft gel capsules per day with meals)
- Mobility 2 (2 to 4 tablets three times per day) to reduce inflammation, plus Clear Heat (2 to 3 tablets three to four times per day) if heat signs
- Power Mushrooms (3 tablets three times per day) is used between flare-ups to improve immune functioning
- Nine Flavor Tea (3 tablets three times per day) as an adjunct formula with dry eyes, afternoon fever, and other signs of yin deficiency

Rocky Mountain Spotted Fever

Rocky Mountain spotted fever is caused by Rickettsia rickettsii, a bacteria that is spread to humans via tick bites. Its name is a bit of a misnomer, because it is found throughout the continental U.S., as well as in Canada, Mexico, and Central America. Early symptoms such as fever, nausea, vomiting, muscle pain, and lack of appetite appear five to ten days after a tick bite. A flat, pink rash may appear two to five days after the fever, though the characteristic red, spotted rash doesn't appear until after six days or more. Rocky Mountain spotted fever can be a very serious illness, and because it infects cells lining the blood vessels, can involve all the body's systems. Antibiotics should be administered immediately when Rocky Mountain spotted fever is suspected, with doxycycline as the drug of choice.

Professional Treatment

♦ Clear Heat (2 to 3 tablets three to four times per day) can be administered if antibiotics do not seem to work. Clear Heat can be applied as a wash
♦ Probiotics to offset damage caused by antibiotics

Scleroderma

In scleroderma, which literally means "hard skin," too much collagen collects in the body. In addition to a thickening and tightening of the skin, there may be joint pain and stiffness, and swelling of the hands and feet in the morning. Scleroderma is thought to be either an autoimmune disease or a blood vessel deficit that causes excessive collagen buildup. Raynaud's phenomenon—in which the skin of the fingers turns from white to blue to pinkish following exposure to cold or stress—is common in scleroderma patients. In some cases, hypertension, kidney failure, lung complications, and intestinal problems are also seen. Exercise is often recommended to help reduce stiffness and to improve blood flow. It is also recommended that you quit smoking, and that you keep your body, especially your hands and feet, warm at all times. Medications depend on the signs and symptoms. For example, blood dilators are used if Raynaud's is present, analgesics are used for pain, and drugs may be used to reduce blood pressure.

Self-Help

♦ Fish oil containing EPA/DHA (3 to 10 g. per day), cod-liver oil (1 to 3 tsp. per day), or EPAQ krill oil (3 soft gel capsules per day with meals)

- High-potency antioxidant such as Quercenol (use as directed)
- Gotu kola (1,000 to 4,000 mg. per day)
- Vitamin E (400 to 800 IU per day)

Professional Treatment

- Collagenex is used to improve skin elasticity and for joint pain (4 tablets per day)
- Mobility 2 and Flavonex (2 tablets of each formula four times per day) to reduce stiffness and improve blood flow
- Resinall K: mix 1 part Resinall K with 3 parts safflower oil and apply topically 2 to 3 times a day
- If in cold condition, add hot ginger compress: add powdered ginger to boiling water for five minutes, steep ten minutes, apply to washcloth, then massage into skin

Sinus Infection

Sinus infection is characterized by difficulty breathing through the nose, pain around the nose, cheeks, and eyes, and fever. The infection may be bacterial, viral, or fungal. Chronic hay fever (allergic rhinitis) can cause sinusitis, because infections can form in the mucus in the nose and spread to the sinus. Other causes include the common cold, a deviated septum, and dental abscess.

Acute sinusitis is usually caused by a bacterial infection, while chronic sinusitis is the result of repeated or untreated acute infections, which may also cause a fungal infection. Diagnosis is made on the basis of symptoms and a laboratory culture. X-rays and CT scans may also be indicated for recurrent sinusitis. Antibiotics or anti-fungal medications may be recommended. Herbal remedies are particularly helpful for recurrent infections, or for infections that aren't satisfactorily treated with antibiotics.

Self-Help

- Water helps thin mucus, so drinking plenty of fluids will help you recover
- Warm water compresses or inhaling steam several times a day. (Place several drops of eucalyptus, oregano, or white flower oil in a pot of boiling water. Take off stove, cover your head with a towel, and inhale the vapors, being careful not to get burned.) A more high-tech solution is steam inhaler devices
- High potency antioxidant such as Quercenol (use as directed)
- Irrigating the sinus twice per day can be very helpful. Use products that are already prepared or mix 1/3 tsp. table salt in 8 oz. warm water. You can add 1/3 tsp. baking soda as desired. Spray into each nostril while closing off the other and simultaneously inhaling. A few drops of goldenseal tincture may be added for its anti-fungal effects

Professional Treatment

- Phellostatin (3 tablets three times per day)
- Nasal Tabs 2 (2 to 3 tablets three to four times per day); add Coptis Purge Fire with heat signs including colored phlegm
- Flavonex (2 to 3 tablets three times per day) for circulation, long term for clients who have damaged nasal mucosa; add Resinall E short term to improve healing response

- ◆ Power Mushrooms (1 to 3 tablets three times per day) to improve immune system

Case Study

Reiner was a fifty-two-year-old travel writer. While visiting Asia he developed an acute sinus infection, although he often had signs of chronic sinusitis as well as allergic rhinitis (hay fever) aggravated by pollution. His doctor prescribed the antibiotic amoxicillin for two weeks. Within a few days of stopping the antibiotic, the infection returned. He went to a different doctor, who prescribed a different antibiotic, a steroid nasal spray, and pseudoephedrine HCl. After finishing this protocol, all the symptoms returned. When we saw him, he was experiencing headaches over the forehead, congestion, postnasal drip with yellow-green phlegm, and reduced sense of smell. His tongue was red with a dark yellow thin coat, and his pulse was slippery. We recommended Nasal Tabs 2 (2 tablets four times per day) with Coptis Purge Fire (2 tablets four times per day) and goldenseal tincture (2 drops per application) added to an over-the-counter saline spray every two hours. In his next appointment in two weeks, all symptoms were eliminated. Reiner had said the sinuses felt better after three days, and after a week the symptoms were totally eliminated. His tongue was red, and his pulse was less slippery. We recommended a follow-up protocol of Phellostatin (2 tablets three times per day), which has anti-fungal and tonifying effects.

Discussion: Nasal Tabs 2 contains several herbs for opening sinuses and also increasing blood circulation, which is necessary due to damage caused by congestion. Coptis Purge Fire is a strong heat-clearing formula that has anti-fungal and antibiotic properties, although in a much broader spectrum fashion than pharmaceuticals. Nasal irrigation is important, as it applies saline, anti-fungal and anti-bacterial herbs to the sinus directly.

Recent research at the Mayo Clinic has revealed that single or multiple fungal infections are involved in most chronic sinus infections. The most common fungi found were candida, aspergillus, cladosporium, and penicillin species. There may also simultaneously exist a bacterial infection as well as an allergic response to the fungus.

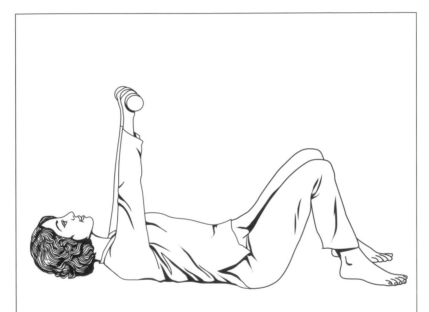

Flat Press
Lie face up on a bench with your feet planted on the floor on either side, or lie down on the floor with your knees bent and your feet flat on the floor. With your elbows bent and close to your body, hold a weight in each hand, about an inch over your armpits. Your palms should face the ceiling. Slowly press both weights upward until your arms are fully extended and the insides of your elbows face each other. Bring the weights toward each other, allowing the ends to touch over your chest. Pause at the top, and then slowly separate the weights and lower them toward your armpits. Do 12–15 repetitions per set, complete three sets.

Sjögren's Syndrome

Sjögren's syndrome is an autoimmune disease in which lymphocytes attack moisture-producing glands, causing dryness in the mouth and eyes particularly, but also in the rest of the body. It's characterized by symptoms like dry skin and rashes, joint and muscle pain, numbness and tingling in the extremities, thyroid problems, and pneumonia. Sjögren's is also a rheumatic disease, and so can cause inflammation throughout the body. Because the symptoms of Sjögren's syndrome are similar to those of many other diseases, diagnosis can take years. Diagnosis is positive with symptoms of dry mouth and eyes, and a positive biopsy of minor salivary glands on the lower lip. Blood tests for antibodies associated with Sjögren's can identify other parts of the body that may be affected. Dryness symptoms are treated with artificial tears and saliva stimulants such as pilocarpine and cevimeline. NSAIDs are used for joint and muscle pain, and corticosteroids and immunosuppressants such as hydroxychloroquine, methotrexate, and cyclophosphamide are used for symptoms in the organs, blood vessels, and nervous system.

Self-Help

◆ Keep a humidifier in the rooms where you spend the most time.

Professional Treatment

◆ Nine Flavor Tea (3 tablets three times per day) to reduce dryness

- EPAQ krill oil (3 soft gel capsules per day with meals) has anti-inflammatory effects and helps the body produce moisture
- Mobility 2 (2 to 4 tablets three times per day) to reduce inflammation, plus Clear Heat (2 to 3 tablets three to four times per day) if heat signs

Thyroid Disorders

The thyroid secretes the hormones thyroxine (T4) and tri-iodothyronine (T3), which regulate the body's metabolism. When the thyroid makes too much thyroid hormone, it's called *hyperthyroidism*. Too much thyroid hormone speeds up the metabolism, causing anxiety, restlessness, insomnia, weight loss, increased heart rate, high blood pressure, nervousness, diarrhea, muscle weakness, trembling hands, menstrual problems, and bulging eyeballs. Hyperthyroidism is most commonly caused by Graves' disease, an autoimmune disorder that inappropriately causes the thyroid to produce too many hormones. A diagnosis is based on an increased heart rate, possibly enlarged thyroid, elevated blood levels of T3 and T4, and decreased blood levels of TSH (thyroid-stimulating hormone). Hyperthyroidism is treated with anti-thyroid medications, which can have serious side effects; or radioactive iodine or surgery, both of which can result in hypothyroidism. Hyperthyroidism may also be caused by thyroid tumors that produce excess hormones.

When the thyroid doesn't make enough hormones, it's called *hypothyroidism*. When there's not enough thyroid hormone, the body slows down—producing lethargy, fatigue, depression, slower heart rate, constipation, weight gain, increased sensitivity to cold, and numbness in the hands. Hypothyroidism is most commonly caused by Hashimoto's thyroiditis, an autoimmune condition in which antibodies damage the thyroid, which in turn doesn't produce enough thyroid hormone. Hypothyroidism may also be caused by too much iodine. A positive thyroid autoimmune antibody test indicates Hashimoto's thyroiditis. Hashimoto's thyroiditis, like any hypothyroid condition, is treated with thyroid hormone replacement drugs. Many natural practitioners prefer natural Armour thyroid to synthetic Synthroid.

Professional Treatment

- For mild *hyperthyroidism:* Nine Flavor Tea (3 tablets three times per day), add Calm Spirit (3 tablets three times per day) with anxiety or Clear Heat (2 to 3 tablets three to four times per day) with heat signs
- For *hypothyroidism:* Rehmannia 8 (3 tablets three times per day) long term. Adrenosen (2 to 3 tablets three times per day) may be added

Trichomoniasis

Trichomoniasis is a vaginal infection caused by *Trichomonas vaginalis,* a sexually transmitted parasite. Symptoms in women include a frothy, foul-smelling green or yellowish vaginal discharge, itching of the vagina, labia, and inner thighs, and discomfort with intercourse. While men may be infected too, their infection often has no symptoms and goes away on its own in a few weeks. Trichomoniasis is treated with antibiotics, commonly metronidazole (Flagyl).

Professional Treatment

◆ Artestatin (2 to 3 tablets three times per day) can be used if antibiotics are not effective

Tuberculosis (TB)

Tuberculosis has been known since antiquity, but didn't reach epidemic proportions until 19th century England, where it spread in crowded, urban slums. TB is a chronic bacterial infection spread by inhaling infected air. TB bacteria typically grow in the lungs, causing a bad cough that lasts longer than two weeks, coughing up blood or sputum, pain in the chest, weakness and fatigue, loss of weight and appetite, chills, fever, and sweating at night.

Once the leading cause of death in the U.S., TB had almost disappeared after the 1940s, when drugs were discovered that could treat it. In Africa and Asia, however, TB has consistently been a major cause of death. And while early detection and public awareness brought about a decline of TB in Europe and the U.S. in the 20th century, TB has made a comeback in recent years, the result of a confluence of factors including decreased funding for public health TB-control programs, antibiotic resistance, IV drug use, and AIDS. In the U.S. today, TB remains a problem for infants, drug users, seniors, and people with weak immune systems. Each year worldwide, 54 million people are infected with TB, 6.8 million develop the disease, and 2.4 million die from it. TB is the leading cause of death for people with HIV, and development of TB is an early sign of immunosuppression in HIV-positive individuals.

Diagnosis of TB is made on the basis of the tuberculin skin test and chest X-rays, as well as by examining and testing your sputum. A combination of antibiotics is typically prescribed for

TB, such as isoniazid, rifampin, pyrazinamide, streptomycin, and ethambutol. Side effects may include nausea, vomiting, and abnormal liver function. Isoniazid is given as a preventive for family members and health care workers whose skin tests are positive for TB, but whose X-ray is negative. In this case, the benefits of the antibiotic must be weighed against its toxicity. In the past, people with TB were isolated, but this is no longer necessary beyond a few days as long as medication is taken. Natural remedies can be used as adjuncts to standard care.

Professional Treatment

- CordySeng (2 tablets two to three times per day) to improve oxygen capacity
- Tremella & American Ginseng (3 to 5 tablets four times per day) with dry cough and heat signs

Urinary Tract Infection/Cystitis

Urinary tract infections (UTI), also called cystitis, affect the kidney, bladder, or urethra. They are very common among women. Sexual activity, pregnancy, and urinary blockage can cause bacteria to multiply. Some bacteria are so strong they cannot be flushed out by urine.

Cystitis is characterized by frequent and urgent urination, burning, bloody, or smelly urine, and lower abdominal discomfort or pressure. Although sexually active women are most likely to get cystitis, it also occurs because the anus is so close to the urethra—90 percent of cystitis cases are due to E. coli, bacteria found in the rectal area. If you have symptoms of cystitis, visit your health professional. Your urine may need to be analyzed, and antibiotics are usually administered. It is common practice to administer antibiotics continuously to women who have frequent UTIs, which may predispose clients to yeast infections and antibiotic resistance.

Urethritis produces frequent and painful urination, with pus in the urine and discharge from the penis. In women, there may be sexually transmitted infections such as herpes simplex and chlamydia, or other bacteria that cause UTIs. In men, urethritis may be caused by sexually transmitted chlamydia and gonorrhea. Because urethritis is often caused by a sexually transmitted disease, antibiotics are usually needed to prevent more serious conditions from occurring.

Kidney infection, or pyelonephritis, is characterized by high fever, chills, vomiting, burning urination and increased urinary frequency. Antibiotics and further diagnostic tests may be administered.

Self-Help

- D–Mannose (½ tsp. four times per day) in initial stage of infection only. D–Mannose is a simple sugar that attaches to E. coli bacteria in the urinary tract and flushes it out in the urine. If it's going to work, it will work quickly.
- Unsweetened cranberry juice (16 oz. per day) or cranberry capsules (use as directed). Compounds found in cranberries are thought to prevent bacteria from sticking to the walls of the urinary tract.
- Probiotics (use as directed)

Professional Treatment

◆ Akebia Moist Heat (3 tablets four to six times per day) at first signs of UTI

◆ Clearing (3 tablets three times per day), use to prevent UTI

Case Study

Sharon was a fourteen-year-old student who had been on antibiotics for almost a year and a half since visiting our clinic for urinary tract infections and respiratory infections. Although bacteria were not always present, she reported pelvic pain and burning with urination if she stopped taking the antibiotics. Sharon's pulse was soggy, and her tongue was dry and pale, with a yellow coat in the rear of the tongue. We suggested to Sharon's mother that she pursue testing for fungus, as fungus can cause UTI, and can also be spread due to the overuse of antibiotics. Sharon had tried cranberry juice without success in the past.

We recommended PB8 acidophilus (2 capsules two times per day) to replenish good bacteria, and Phellostatin (2 tablets three times per day) as a natural anti-fungal. Against my suggestion, Sharon's mother took Sharon off her antibiotics and herbs, within a few days Sharon got another UTI, which required her to return to the antibiotics. After two weeks, Sharon's symptoms, pulse, and tongue were unchanged so she resumed her protocol of herbs. After two more weeks her mother had Sharon take antibiotics every other day, while taking the herbs. Her pulse was soggy, and her tongue had lost some of the yellow coating. At this point I recommended adding Drain Dampness *(wu ling san)* (2 tablets three times per day), while maintaining on the PB8 and Phellostatin. After another month of taking antibiotics every other day, Sharon was able to be weaned off antibiotics. In the meantime the family started working with an osteopath. Over the next three months of using the herbs, Sharon has been antibiotic free. During this time we replaced the Phellostatin with the more tonifying Six Gentlemen (3 tablets twice per day), which also reduces dampness.

Vasculitis

Vasculitis is an inflammation of any of the blood vessels in the body, from the tiniest capillaries and venules, to the large vessels supplying major organs. Inflammation leads to scarring, which makes the vessels too narrow for blood to get through to the organs. Symptoms of vasculitis include fatigue, weakness, fever, joint pain, abdominal pain, and kidney and nerve problems. Vasculitis is commonly treated with cortisone or cytotoxic drugs. The following professional treatments should be used as adjuncts to standard approaches.

Professional Treatment

- EPAQ krill oil (3 soft gel capsules per day with meals) for anti-inflammatory effect
- Mobility 2 (2 to 4 tablets three times per day) treats joint pain
- Flavonex (2 to 3 tablets three times per day) promotes circulation and reduces inflammation

Chapter Four

Digestive Clearing Diet

I f your goal is to greatly reduce or eliminate the symptoms of your immune disorder, you must be prepared to examine the foods you are eating. The terms "allergy," "intolerance," and "sensitivity" are used loosely by many people. A *food allergy* actually means that the body's immune system mounts a response to the offending allergen. A true allergy can be diagnosed by laboratory tests, such as with a skin prick or radioallergosorbent test (RAST). Many persons with immune and autoimmune disorders have *food sensitivities* (food intolerance), which cannot be detected by a laboratory test, but must be determined through trial and error. Sensitivities can cause such symptoms as abdominal cramping, diarrhea, constipation, intestinal gas, bloating, vomiting, nausea, ulcers, fatigue, joint pain, muscle aches, edema, headaches, migraines, depression, anxiety, respiratory difficulties, hyperactivity, and attention disorders.

Why are we so sensitive? We are exposed to thousands of chemicals our ancestors were never exposed to: pollutants, residues from fertilizer and pesticides, additives, preservatives, and flavoring agents, among others. The earliest nutritionist was our nose and tongue. The foods we needed smelled good; when we had enough to eat, the food no longer appealed to our taste. With the advent of food processing, our senses of taste and smell were no longer reliable. And when the refrigerator and modern transportation came into being, foods that are genetically intolerable became available.

Our ancestors ate what was available in their environments. The Native American Indian of the Plains who was severely allergic to buffalo, the Asian who couldn't eat rice, or the Irish who couldn't eat potatoes, simply died. People then were much more active, so sensitivities were not taken into consideration. Every day was a struggle for survival. When chased by wild animals, or fighting a warring tribe, one does not concern oneself about abdominal pain or constipation!

It is no wonder that millions of us have digestive and immune disorders. We are bombarded with stress and don't exercise, we are exposed to foods and chemicals our digestive systems weren't designed to handle, and many of us were not breast-fed. Breast-feeding seems to protect us from developing allergies and sensitivities. Another problem that people face is food cravings. Often, the cravings are for foods that one is actually sensitive to. I have counseled many digestive and respiratory patients who make statements like: "I must have cereal and milk every morning." Parts of the treatment involve refraining from the food one craves, in this case cereal and milk, for at least two weeks. Other unhealthy cravings may be dairy, alcohol, fruit, sweets, fructose, tomatoes, soy, and greasy foods. When the food cravings are based on emotional difficulties, psychological counseling may also be helpful.

Digestive Meal Plan

The purpose of the digestive clearing meal plan is to help you identify foods that are problematic for your body. If you follow this plan faithfully you can greatly reduce or eliminate your digestive and immune symptoms. You should plan about one month for your digestive clearing program. I recommend that you do not begin when holidays, vacations, or celebrations are planned. It is very much like quitting smoking: you need to make a plan.

It is possible that you may feel worse for the first few days of clearing, but don't cheat! It will be worth it in the long run. As I do not believe in making drastic changes, the first two weeks are a "winding down" period; the next two weeks consist of taking in foods that are not commonly known to cause sensitivities, followed by a reintroduction phase. It is essential that you keep a journal during this process. Once you have located a food you are sensitive to, it may be possible through the use of herbs and other dietary supplements to build up your system so that you can occasionally incorporate it back into your diet. You may notice that you feel so much better without consuming a formerly craved food, that it is not worthwhile to reincorporate it. Chapter One has a list of foods that have been known to produce reactions in digestive patients.

For the first two weeks, you should begin reducing and then eliminating "not allowed" foods from your diet. If you are eating any of these foods more than once a day, you should cut down your consumption by 50 percent the first day, then eliminate it by the end of the second week. All food you eat should be cooked. This will reduce food reactivity. Locate a health food store or supermarket where you can obtain fresh foods and foods without additives, pesticides, antibiotics, and hormones. Drink at least 64 oz. of filtered or spring water, or herbal teas. You may place a slice of cucumber, lemon, or lime wedge in the water to make it tastier. You should maintain the increased water or herbal tea intake throughout the clearing and reintroduction phase. Whenever possible, drink hot water; *never drink ice water.* If taken from the refrigerator, let water reach room temperature.

I have provided a sample meal plan below. Feel free to improvise as long as you are eating the allowable foods. The not-allowed list is not exhaustive, so if the food is not on the allowed list, don't eat it! Also included are recommendations for the use of supplements, which should be started during the preparation phase, or after clearing is completed.

Protein

Allowed
Beef, pork, lamb, venison, chicken, turkey, duck, goose, rabbit, pheasant, quail, or other game. Fresh fish.

Not Allowed
Shellfish, prepared fish (such as breaded fish or fish sticks), prepared or preserved meats (such as bacon, sausages, hot dogs, cold cuts).

Preparation
Boiled, baked, broiled, and poached. Avoid deep frying.

Vegetables

Allowed
Most. Limit potatoes to 1 per day.

Not Allowed

Soybean, tomatoes, cabbage, broccoli, cauliflower, mushrooms, brussels sprouts, beans, peas, lentils. These should be the first foods to be reintroduced.

Preparation

Try to use only fresh vegetables. Frozen vegetables may be used when in a pinch. All vegetables should be steamed or boiled. Light stir-frying with olive oil is suitable. Spray olive oil or use a maximum of 1 Tbsp. per serving of extra virgin olive oil. After two weeks begin to use salads with olive, canola, hemp, or flax oils (no more than 1 Tbsp. of oil per serving). Add vinegar a few days later.

Fruits

Allowed

None during the digestive clearing phase. Thereafter, begin with bananas, pears, apples, kiwifruit, mangoes, papaya, pomegranates, passion fruit, guava, and melons. Blueberries, strawberries, raspberries, and other fruit may be added later, after you have tested the previous fruits.

Starch and Grains

Allowed

Rice, millet, amaranth, tapioca, buckwheat, and quinoa. During the reintroduction phase, add gluten-containing foods (oats, barley, rye, spelt), and yeast-free muffins and crackers before adding breads.

Nuts

Eliminate during the clearing phase. During the reintroduction phase, you can start incorporating nuts and nut butters; however, peanuts and peanut butter should be tested last (technically, peanuts are legumes).

Seasoning

Allowed
Sea salt, pepper, herbs, and spices, if they are used alone (that is, don't use combination seasonings).

Beverages

Allowed
Filtered water, spring water, and herbal tea. Only black or green tea may be used during the preparation phase to reduce or eliminate caffeine cravings. During the reintroduction phase, you can experiment with carbonated water if desired. Fruit juices should be reintroduced last and should be used only half strength or more diluted.

Prohibited Foods

Any food not on the above list, including but not limited to dairy products (milk, cream, butter, cheese, yogurt, ice cream), eggs, sweets, yeast, pastries, prepared or instant food, vinegar, Marmite (yeast extract), alcoholic beverages, canned foods, horseradish, bouillon, bread, bagels, pizza, rolls, chips, salad dressing, desserts, fruits and fruit juices, ice drinks, soda, and uncooked foods.

If You Still Have Symptoms

The digestive clearing plan gives your body a vacation. Not all vacations are great 100 percent of the time. However, when we look back, we can say it was worth it. Therefore, it is realistic to expect withdrawal symptoms for the first few days. For example, on a vacation you may miss your friends or colleagues from work. Similarly, on the clearing plan, you may miss your morning cup of coffee or your gooey sweet roll. If after a week you do not feel fewer symptoms and more energy and mental clarity, it is possible that you could have sensitivities to foods allowed on the digestive clearing diet. If you have eliminated all the items listed as not allowed, try meats that you have not eaten before. The same applies to vegetables. Also, have you been cheating? Check your food diary. Is there something that you ate on the run? One of my clients, Jessica, was not experiencing any improvement on the clearing program; it turns out she had not given up alcohol.

It is also possible that chemicals such as perfume, airplane glue, sprays, lighter fluid, or even particle board may be causing your symptoms. In this case, you should consult a health professional specializing in environmental allergies. In addition, changes in barometric pressure, particularly as the weather becomes more humid, have been known to trigger joint pain and other symptoms.

An elimination diet of lamb, pears, yams, sweet potatoes, millet, rice, and hypoallergenic protein powder (available from holistic health professionals) can be used as an alternative to the digestive clearing plan; however, professional supervision is recommended. Another diet known as the Rare Foods Diet can be selected. This involves eating only foods you have never eaten before, such as ostrich, quinoa, amaranth, and other exotic foods.

Meal Plan with Supplementation

One-half hour before meals take an acidophilus/bifidus product in capsule or powder form. Take a separate product with FOS. Follow instructions on the bottle carefully.

One-half hour before breakfast

◆ Acidophilus/bifidus/FOS

Breakfast

◆ Rice or millet porridge
◆ Antioxidant vitamin, folic acid, and B$_{12}$

Snack

◆ Sweet potato, yam, acorn squash, artichoke, rice cakes

One-half hour before lunch

◆ Acidophilus/bifidus/FOS

Lunch

◆ Homemade beef, chicken, or turkey vegetable soup
◆ Meat or fish
◆ Steamed vegetables and rice
◆ Antioxidant vitamin, folic acid, and B_{12}

Snack

◆ Sweet potato, yam, acorn squash, artichoke, rice cakes

One-half hour before dinner

◆ Acidophilus/bifidus/FOS

Dinner

◆ Meat, fish, or homemade soup
◆ Vegetable—steamed, boiled, or stir-fried (1 Tbsp. extra virgin olive oil per serving)
◆ Allowable grains
◆ Sweet potato, yam, acorn squash
◆ Pasta made from quinoa or Jerusalem artichoke

Beverages

- Filtered water
- Herbal tea: Pau D'Arco, peppermint, ginger (with cold signs), most other herbal teas

Bedtime

- Acidophilus/bifidus/FOS
- Healing bath (see Chapter One, "Tips for a Healthy Immune System")

Reintroduction Phase

After two weeks, begin reintroducing foods in the indicated order. A new food can be introduced every four hours. If symptoms occur, put that food on your list of items to be tested at a later date. If you were under stress, fatigued, or menstruating when testing, put on your "possible sensitivity" list and retest in one month or so. Start with the vegetables indicated. See if raw or cooked makes a difference, starting with one to two serving of vegetables per day. If this agrees with you, try making homemade oil and herb dressing. If this agrees with you, add vinegar in a few days.

Next, introduce whole fruit, then oatmeal, yeast-free muffins, followed by crackers, then by all other foods. Put off processed foods and multi-ingredient foods as long as possible, as they make identifying sensitivities more difficult. If you follow this plan under the guidance of a health professional, he or she may suggest protein powders and added nutrients. There are pros and cons of adding vitamins to this program. In general, if you can, high-quality, hypoallergenic vitamins are recommended. They will help you heal your gastrointestinal system faster (see Chapter Two). The disadvantage of using vitamins at this point is that they may mask symptoms, but I believe that the advantages of vitamins far outweigh this one disadvantage.

If constipation occurs while undergoing this program, supplement ground flax seeds, flax oil, guar gum, and other soluble fibers. You can also increase your consumption of vegetables and add prunes. If your stools are looser while following this program, temporarily reduce the vegetables (and fruits, if you are into the reintroduction phase) and introduce them more slowly. If you are still having problems, seek the help of a health professional.

I have personally found this plan to be very beneficial. My clients and other health professionals agree that giving their digestive systems a break is very helpful. Admittedly, it is more difficult for vegetarians. It may be possible to obtain protein in the form of protein shakes. However, many of these products have common allergens and contain ingredients such as algae and spirulina that are hard to digest. Hypoallergenic protein powders can be obtained through holistic professionals.

Digestive Clearing Worksheet

This worksheet is to help you identify your food sensitivities.

- What foods can't I live without?

_____

_____

- What foods lead to symptoms, or do I suspect I may be sensitive to? (Do not edit.)

_____

_____

_____

- What major dietary change have I undertaken? Did that make my digestion better or worse?

  _____

  _____

- What foods or beverages do I have more than once per day?

  _____

  _____

- What do I like to do that does not involve eating?

  _____

  _____

Chapter Five

Commonly Asked Questions and Answers

◆ *Is it safe to use antioxidant herbs and supplements with chemotherapy?*

Many cancer therapies work by producing free radicals; therefore, some doctors have voiced concerns about using antioxidants, which reduce free radicals. There is very little evidence from the scientific literature that supports this concern. In fact, some studies have shown that antioxidants improved the cancer therapy. Drug antioxidants such as amifostine and mesna have been studied with chemotherapy and radiation, and have not caused a negative reaction. In a fifty-two patient trial, the antioxidant glutathione was combined with oxaliplatin,[1] a chemotherapy drug. Patients taking the antioxidant had a lower incidence of chemo-induced nerve damage than those taking the placebo. Furthermore, the glutathione did not reduce the effects of the chemo, and patients taking glutathione showed slightly more tumor shrinkage than those who did not use glutathione. Vitamins

C and E, carotenes, milk thistle, and ginkgo are popular antioxidants.

◆ *My doctor says there's no science or little science behind herbal remedies. Is this true?*

On one hand, your doctor is right, except for a few superstar herbs such as soy, astragalus, ginseng, echinacea, saw palmetto, modified citrus pectin, milk thistle, bilberry, tang kuei, green tea, and huperzine A. From an empirical standpoint it could be argued that herbs that have been used for hundreds of years are better researched than pharmaceutical drugs.

◆ *I went to a practitioner of Chinese medicine once and it didn't help me. How do I know it isn't all hype?*

There are many aspects of Chinese medicine. The two most popular in the West are acupuncture and Chinese herbs. In general, if you have a serious health problem, it is not realistic that you would have lasting improvement after one session. For people with cancer or other serious immune problems, several months of treatment are required as a minimum. Keep in mind that Chinese medicine is very subjective. Some practitioners are better than others. Some practitioners get better results with certain patients or conditions. It sounds like you needed to give it more time, and or find a practitioner you like better.

◆ *My friend was diagnosed with breast cancer. She has decided to go "all natural" and has decided to treat herself with raw juices and vitamins. Do you think this is a good idea?*

No. I think if you live in the U.S. you should avail yourself of the best biomedical and the best complementary methods in combination. Each by itself has limitations. In many cases catching the disease early, being able to conduct precision surgery, using herbs, and the judicious use of dietary supplements may produce the best possible results. Even if the cancer is caught later, the herbs and vitamins can greatly help reduce chemotherapy and radiation side effects, and may help prevent cancer recurrence. On one hand, juicing is good in that it provides easy-to-digest nutrients; on the other hand, drinking a lot of raw juices can be too cooling for many constitutional types.

◆ *Is there any way to predict whether or not I will be able to tolerate an herbal product or a nutritional supplement?*

People who are fearful, emotionally exhausted, and underweight, and have low blood pressure or are in poor health tend to be more sensitive than other people. If one or all of these apply, you might consider taking a reduced dosage of all herbs and supplements, at least for the first week or two, in order to see if you can tolerate a particular product. Keep in mind that quality as well as additives and binders can also impact the tolerability. In

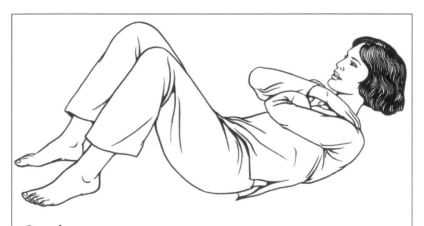

Crunch
Lie on your back with your knees bent, and your feet flat on the floor. Fold your arms across your chest. Lift your shoulders a few inches off the floor, toward your hipbones, to help curl your upper spine forward. Pause, then slowly lower your shoulders to the floor. Do 12–15 repetitions per set, complete three sets.

some cases, people think they are intolerant to the herb or vita-min, when they are really reacting to an additive or binder. On the other hand, if you have severe allergies such as anaphylactic shock to an item such as seafood or peanuts, it makes sense to avoid it altogether.

◆ *What is the difference between celiac disease, gluten intolerance, and wheat allergy?*

Celiac disease is a particular disease in which gluten proteins damage the intestines. One definition of gluten intolerance that I like is when someone cannot tolerate wheat and other gluten-containing foods, but there is not visible damage to the intestines. Wheat allergy refers to someone who can tolerate certain gluten-containing foods, but cannot tolerate wheat in any form. These clients will typically do best having no more than a few servings per week of alternative gluten foods such as spelt and kamut.

◆ *Aren't individualized teas or tinctures always best?*

In many communities there are herbal healers who put together their own formulas in the form of teas or tinctures. Some of these healers are very gifted. On the other hand, many of the traditional healers do not have knowledge of herb-drug interac-tions or modern quality-control issues. Therefore, if these are concerns of yours, it may be better to go to an herbalist who uses prepackaged products, where the ingredients are clearly marked on the label, and there is accountability regarding the quality of herbal ingredients.

◆ *My client had radiation five times a week for two months for cancer treatment. Nothing I have tried helped his fatigue. What do you sug-gest?*

Power Mushrooms will help deal with the fatigue (2-3 tablets two to three times per day). If you think about it, his body has

310

been subjected to a bombardment not unlike bombing used in warfare. Just as it takes some time after bombing to build back the houses; it will take time to get his energy back. Herbs such as Power Mushrooms will only help him; however, he might be too weak or in too much pain to notice any difference right now. The difference will be more apparent in four to six weeks, particularly if he remains on the herbs.

◆ *I have had a long-standing immune problem. The doctors recommend long-term antibiotics and steroids, although it was recently recommended that I go on a new experimental drug. Having been unsuccessfully treated by an M.D. who specializes in acupuncture and Chinese medicine, I am wary of herbs and alternative medicine, yet I don't want to take these drugs forever. What should I do?*

If you go to a doctor and they don't help you, most people find a different doctor. One should not rule out all of alternative medicine on the basis of one practitioner. The same is true with herbal medicine. If you try an herbal formula dispensed by one practitioner and it doesn't work, either find a different herbalist, or request that your herbal provider change your herbal protocol.

In terms of getting off medication, this would be recommended only after you have found an alternative approach that works best for you, and after you have weighed the pros and cons with your health professional. It is essential that you have a plan for slowly getting off your prescription drugs. Generally the longer you have been on medication, the more time it may take to get off it.

◆ *I only want to use alternatives that have been proven in well-designed research studies. What proof is there that herbs work?*

First of all, the proof that herbs work is that they have been used continually for hundreds if not thousands of years. This is particularly the case with traditional Chinese herbal medicine, which has done an enormous job in preserving herbal heritage. Although Western-style research has been conducted on herbs, for the most part it is done in Europe and Asia and much of it has not been translated into English. From the standpoint of empirical knowledge, traditional Chinese medicine is the world's second most common form of medicine; it is used by a billion Chinese and Westerners. Millions of patients visit acupuncturists; in the U.S. many licensed acupuncturists are trained in herbology. Chinese medicine has continued to evolve over the last two thousand years from diseases caused by colds, SARS, and protocols that help people undergoing chemo and radiotherapy.

In terms of "well-designed research studies," it is important to realize that by and large, research is not used by individual M.D.s to make treatment decisions. Treatment decisions are based upon each individual doctor's clinical experience and also on the basis of fashion, marketing, and feedback from other practitioners. Currently, multi-drug treatment is widely recommended by doctors to treat immune and other conditions, but the odds are extremely small that the same combination of drugs you are on is well researched. As Western medicine as it is practiced is not research-driven, why would you hold alternatives to a higher standard?

Hopefully, one day more research can be focused on studying drug prescriptions the way they are administered clinically, and on subjecting herbs to more clinical trials. If you wait for that date to occur, you may be missing out on many important breakthroughs, but that is your choice.

◆ *I have an autoimmune condition. Couldn't herbs and supplements that are supposed to bolster the immune system make me worse?*

At our clinic and our affiliated clinics we have been administering herbs to immune-compromised individuals for two decades. Some of these individuals have AIDS and other serious autoimmune conditions. It is our clinical experience that well-designed, high-quality herbs and supplements help many of these individuals. As the autoimmune phenomenon really means the immune system is not working well, by improving immune functioning, the body is less likely to attack itself. In addition, herbs and supplements can be used to reduce infections, which down-regulate the immune system even further.

♦ *My doctor said not to take herbs because they interact with drugs.*

Certain herbs like St. John's wort do seem to interact with many medications, but it is not proven that all herbs interact with medication. There are a few guidelines to keep in mind when you are taking medication and want to add supplements and herbs. First, always take herbs and drugs two hours apart. Second, find an herbalist or another health professional who can guide you as to which herbs may be safe and which herbs to avoid. Finally, it is a good idea not to go off any pharmaceutical medication without consulting your health professional.

Appendix A

Additional Formulas

Following are the formulas not elaborated on in Chapter Two, their applications, and their ingredients.

Adrenosen™

Typical Applications: Tonify adrenals, pituitary, thyroid; energy tonic

Chinese Therapeutic Actions: Tonify Qi and kidney yang, drain dampness

Ingredients: Adrenal cortex, PAK *(pyridoxal alpha ketoglutarate)*, Pseudostellaria root *(tai zi shen)*, Dioscorea root *(shan yao)*, Dolichos seed *(bai bian dou)*, Schizandra fruit *(wu wei zi)*, Oryza sprout *(gu ya)*

Akebia Moist Heat™

Typical Applications: Urinary tract infections; cystitis

Chinese Therapeutic Actions: Clear fire and toxins in lower burner, drain dampness

Ingredients: Akebia Trifoliata Caulis *(mu tong)*, Pyrossia leaf *(shi wei)*, Plantago seed *(che qian zi)*, Dianthus herb *(qu mai)*, Lygodium spore *(hai jin shu)*, Gardenia fruit *(zhi zi)*, Talcum *(hua shi)*, Soft Russ pith *(deng xing cao)*, Licorice root *(gan cao)*, Vladimiria Souliei root *(mu xiang)*, Rhubarb rhizome (wine steamed) *(zhi da huang)*

Antler 8

Typical Applications: Blood deficiency, deficient immune functions, impotence, knee arthralgia

Chinese Therapeutic Actions: Nourish marrow, generate blood, invigorate yang

Ingredients: Deer Antler *(lu rong)*, Salvia *(dan shen)*, Rehmannia *(di huang)*, Polygonatum *(huang jing)*, Ginseng *(ren shen)*, Tang Kuei *(dang gui)*, Alpinia *(yi zhi ren)*, Cardamon *(sha ren)*

Aquilaria 22™

Typical Applications: Chronic infestations of intestinal parasites; constipation

Chinese Therapeutic Actions: Anti-parasitic, purge gallbladder heat, disperse stagnant Qi, astringe the intestines

Ingredients: Aquilaria sinensis wood (*chen xiang*), Ginger rhizome (*gan jiang*), Mume fruit (*wu mei*), Codonopsis root (*dang shen*), Terminalia fruit (*he zi*), Poria sclerotium (*fu ling*), White Atractylodes rhizome (*bai zhu*), Quisqualis fruit (*shi jun zi*), Omphalia sclerotium (*lei wan*), Vladimiria souliei root (*mu xiang*), Torreya seed (*fei zi*), Areca peel (*da fu pi*), Pomegranate rind (*shi liu pi*), Melia fruit (*chuan lian zi*), Rubus fruit (*fu pen zi*), Aurantium fruit (*zhi shi*), Nutmeg seed (*rou dou kou*), White Cardamon fruit (*bai dou kou*), Ulmus fruit (*wu yi*), Zanthoxylum fruit (*chuan jiao*), Licorice root (*gan cao*), Aloe vera herb (*lu hui*)

Artestatin™

This formula is made up of several anti-parasitic herbs, including artemisia annua (*qing hao*) and the special ingredient brucea, which kills amoebae in the cyst stage. Artestatin is used alone to treat protozoal infections such as giardiasis. For a broader spectrum effect, combine Artestatin with Aquilaria 22, the general dosage being 1 to 3 tablets of Artestatin three times per day and 1 to 2 tablets of Aquilaria 22 three times per day. For diarrhea, decrease the dosage of Aquilaria 22, and for constipation, increase Aquilaria 22.

Typical Applications: Acute infestations of giardia and other protozoa; dysentery, diarrhea

Chinese Therapeutic Actions: Expel parasites, clear summer heat, circulate stagnant Qi, and tonify the spleen and stomach, antimalarial

Ingredients: Artemisia annua concentrate (*qing hao*), Dichroa root (*chang shan*), Brucea fruit (*ya dan zi*), Pulsatilla root (*bai tou weng*), Magnolia bark (*hou po*), Pinellia tuber (*ban xia*), Pogostemon herb

317

(huo xiang), Dolichos seed *(bai bian dou)*, Codonopsis root *(dang shen)*, Citrus peel *(chen pi)*, Licorice root *(gan cao)*, Coptis rhizome *(huang lian)*, Red Atractylodes rhizome *(cang zhu)*, Ginger rhizome *(gan jiang)*, Cardamon fruit *(sha ren)*

Aspiration™

Typical Applications: Mental depression with cold signs

Chinese Therapeutic Actions: Clear stagnant liver qi and blood, remove dampness, resolve food/phlegm entanglement

Ingredients: Polygala root *(yuan zhi)*, Vervain herb (herba verbena officinalis), Uncaria stem *(gou teng)*, Gardenia fruit *(zhi zi)*, Albizzia flowers *(he huan hua)*, Damiana leaf (folium turnerae aphrodisiaciae), White Peony root *(bai shao)*, Tang Kuei *(dang gui)*, Pinellia rhizome *(ban xia)*, Poria sclerotium *(fu ling)*, Aquilaria sinensis wood *(chen xiang)*

Astra C™

Typical Applications: Preventive for colds and flu

Chinese Therapeutic Actions: Strengthen wei qi, relieve the surface

Ingredients: Astragalus root *(huang qi)*, White Atractylodes rhizome *(bai zhu)*, Siler root *(fang feng)*, Rose hips fruit, Acerola, Ascorbic acid, Vitamin C (250 mg.), Zinc Citrate (10 mg.)

Astra Diet Tea™

Typical Applications: To reduce appetite and improve digestion, energy tonic

Chinese Therapeutic Actions: Circulates Qi, tonifies Qi, resolves stomach phlegm, regulates stomach and spleen

Ingredients: Peppermint leaf *(bo he)*, Eleuthero root *(ci wu jia)*, Ginger root *(gan jiang)*, Loquat leaf *(pi pa ye)*, Perilla leaf *(zi su ye)*, Lophatherum leaf *(dan zhu ye)*

Astra Essence™

Typical Applications: Treats degenerative conditions and deterioration of brain function, vertigo, hearing loss, dizziness and loss of memory. Strengthens immune system, an excellent overall tonic and for infertility and impotence. Reduces frequent urination and used to balance glucose in diabetes

Chinese Therapeutic Actions: Tonifies kidney essence (jing), kidney yin and yang, qi and blood

Ingredients: Astragalus root *(huang qi)*, Astragalus seed *(sha yuan ji zi)*, Ligustrum fruit *(nu zhen zi)*, Ho-shou-wu root *(he shou wu)*, Lycium fruit *(gou qi zi)*, Rehmannia (cooked) root *(shu di huang)*, Eucommia bark *(du zhong)*, Cuscuta seed *(tu si zi)*, Ginseng root *(ren shen)*, Tang Kuei root *(dang gui)*, Cornus fruit *(shan zhu yu)*

Backbone™

Typical Applications: Low back pain, bone repair, incontinence, impotence

Chinese Therapeutic Actions: Supplement kidney yang and dispel cold, strengthen sinews/bones, quicken blood and dissipate stasis, strengthen back/knees, secure essence

Ingredients: Eucommia bark *(du zhong),* Psoralea fruit *(bu gu zhi),* Woodwardia orientalis rhizome *(gou ji),* Cuscuta seed *(tu si zi),* Cistanche salsa herb *(rou cong rong),* Rehmannia (cooked) root *(shu di huang),* Tortoise shell (from chinemys reevesii) *(gui ban),* Cyathula root *(chuan niu xi),* Acanthopanax cortex *(wu jia pi),* Tang Kuei Tails root *(dang gui wei),* Dipsacus root *(xu duan),* Carthamus flower *(hong hua),* Myrrh resin *(mo yao),* Cornus fruit *(wu zhu yu)*

Biocidin

Biocidin (Gentiana Formula) is a potent combination of Chinese and Western herbs, including chlorophyll and garlic. It has anti-parasitic, anti-bacterial, and anti-fungal properties. Instructions: during the first week, add 1 to 2 drops of Biocidin to a few ounces of water or juice, or on a cracker with meals. Depending on your tolerance, gradually increase over the course of two to three weeks to 4 to 5 drops. Do not use more than 4 to 5 drops at a time, and do not exceed 15 drops per day total. The average course is six to twelve weeks; however, this may vary accordingly to individual needs. It is not usually necessary to stay at the maximum dosage (15 drops per day) for more than four to eight weeks: a maintenance dosage of 3 to 9 drops total per day should suffice. Biocidin tablets may be taken as directed on the label. This remedy should be taken with the formula Six Gentlemen and aci-dophilus/bifidus supplements. Six Gentlemen counters the cool-ing property of Biocidin, and acidophilus/bifidus restores the health of gut bacteria, which is often disrupted during parasitic infections.

Typical Applications: Candida, parasites, anti-bacterial

Ingredients: Vegetable glycerine, Distilled water, Beet root, Rasp-berry, Milk thistle, Echinacea angustifolia and purpurea, Black Walnut leaf and hull, Noni fruit, Goldenseal, Shiitake, White willow bark, Garlic, Plantain, Fumitory, Gentian, Tea tree oil, Galbanum resin, Lavender oil, Oregano oil, Alcohol

Black Walnut Hulls

Black walnut hulls can be a part of anti-parasitic or anti-worm therapy. I recommend this product be taken in capsule form, starting at 1 capsule per day, up to 5 capsules, three times per day. Some persons report cramping and diarrhea with this herb, so it must be used carefully; however, it may be worth the risk for parasite infections that are not responding to other therapies. An herbalist friend of mine contracted parasites in Indonesia that were drug resistant. After a several-months course of Chinese herbs (Artestatin and Aquilaria 22), she took black walnut hulls in capsule form and was free of the parasites within several months.

Bupleurum Entangled Qi™

Typical Applications: Breast lumps, uterine fibroids/cysts, depres-sion, irritability

Chinese Therapeutic Actions: Vitalize Qi and blood circulation, clear heat and toxins, resolve phlegm

Ingredients: Bupleurum root (*chai hu*), Tang Kuei *(dang gui)*, Blue Citrus fruit *(qing pi)*, Prunella herb *(xia ku cao)*, Salvia root *(dan shen)*, Tricosanthes root *(tian hua fen)*, Vaccaria seed *(wang bu liu xing)*, White Peony root *(bai shao)*, Cyperus rhizome *(xiang fu)*, Ligusticum root *(chuan xiong)*, Fritillaria bulb *(chuan bei mu)*, Tarax-acum herb *(pu gong ying)*, Red Peony root *(chi shao)*

Calm Spirit®

Typical Applications: Stress, anger, anxiety, depression

Chinese Therapeutic Actions: Calm spirit, nourish blood and heart yin, moisten the intestines

Ingredients: Enzymes: Magnesium aspartate, Taurine, Amylase, Cere Calase, Protease, Catalase, Alpha-Galactosidase, Lipase, Glu-coamylase, Cellulase, Malt Diatase; Herbs: Biota seed *(bai zi ren)*, White Peony root *(bai shao)*, Tang Kuei *(dang gui)*, Fu shen scle-rotium *(fu shen)*, Polygala root *(yuan zhi)*, Zizyphus seed *(suan zao ren)*, Ophiopogon tuber *(mai men dong)*, Codonopsis root *(dang shen)*, Amber resin *(hu po)*

Channel Flow™

Typical Applications: Pain-reliever and relaxant; joint, muscle, abdominal, and gynecological pain and cramping; headache, arthritis, and fibromyalgia

Chinese Therapeutic Actions: Regulate Qi and blood, warm the channels

Ingredients: Corydalis extract rhizome *(yan hu suo)*, Angelica root *(bai zhi)*, White Peony root *(bai shao)*, Cinnamon twig *(gui zhi)*, Tang Kuei *(dang gui)*, Salvia root *(dan shen)*, Myrrh resin *(mo yao)*, Frankincense resin *(ru xiang)*, Licorice root *(gan cao)*

Chzyme™

Typical Applications: Taken with meals it will help with food assimilation, reduce intestinal gas, bloating, cramping, regurgitation, nausea, and diarrhea

Chinese Therapeutic Actions: Disperse wind and dampness, resolve spleen dampness and regulate the stomach, resolve phlegm

Ingredients: Amylase, Cere Calase, Protease, Catalase, Alpha-Galactosidase, Lipase, Glucoamylase, Cellulase, Malt Diatase; Herbs: Poria sclerotium *(fu ling)*, Coix seed *(yi yi ren)*, Shen Qu *(shen qu)*, Magnolia bark *(hou po)*, Angelica root *(bai zhi)*, Pueraria root *(ge gen)*, Red Atractylodes rhizome *(cang zhu)*, Vladimiria souliei *(mu xiang)*, Pogostemon herb *(huo xiang)*, Oryza sprout *(gu ya)*, Trichosanthes root *(tian hua fen)*, Chrysanthemum flower *(ju hua)*, Halloysite resin *(chi shi zhi)*, Citrus peel *(ju hong)*, Mentha oil *(bo he)*

Clear Air™

Typical Applications: Asthma, acute/chronic cough; stop-smoking programs

Chinese Therapeutic Actions: Stop cough, dispel phlegm, clear lung

Ingredients: Perilla fruit *(su zi)*, Bai Qian *(bai qian)*, Apricot seed *(ku xing ren)*, Morus cortex *(sang bai pi)*, Tricosanthes root *(tian hua fen)*, Fritillaria bulb *(zhe bei mu)*, Platycodon root *(jie geng)*, Aster root *(zi wan)*, Belamcanda rhizome *(she gan)*, Scute root *(huang qin)*, Schizandra fruit *(wu wei zi)*, Licorice root *(gan cao)*, Pinellia rhizome *(ban xia)*, Tylophora extract leaf

Clear Heat™

Typical Applications: Protocols for viral infections, hepatitis, HIV

Chinese Therapeutic Actions: Clear heat and clean toxins, dissolve phlegm nodules, tonify kidney essence and lung yin

Ingredients: Isatis extract leaf and root *(ban lan gen* and *da qing ye)*, Oldenlandia herb *(bai hua she she cao)*, Lonicera flower *(jin yin hua)*, Prunella herb *(xia ku cao)*, Andrographis herb *(chuan xin lian)*, Laminaria leaf *(kun bu)*, Viola herb/root *(zi hua di ding)*, Cordyceps fruiting body *(dong chong xia cao)*, Licorice root *(gan cao)*

Clear Phlegm™

Typical Applications: Phlegm disorders, expectorant, sedative, bronchitis, nausea, vomiting, dizziness

Chinese Therapeutic Actions: Heat in gallbladder, bitter taste in mouth, phlegm in stomach, slight thirst

Ingredients: Pinellia rhizome *(ban xia)*, Citrus peel *(chen pi)*, Poria sclerotium *(fu ling)*, Aurantium fruit *(zhi shi)*, Bamboo shavings *(zhu ru)*, Arisaema rhizome *(tian nan xing)*, Agastache herb *(huo xiang)*, Acorus rhizome *(shi chang pu)*, Licorice root *(gan cao)*

Clearing™

Typical Applications: Chronic vaginal or urethral irritation, bladder infections

Chinese Therapeutic Actions: Clear heat, tonify spleen, resolve dampness, circulate and nourish the blood

Ingredients: Lotus seed *(lian zi)*, Ophiopogon tuber *(mai men dong)*, Poria sclerotium *(fu ling)*, White Ginseng root *(bai ren shen)*, Plantago seed *(che qian zi)*, Scute root *(huang qin)*, Glehnia root *(sha shen)*, Smilax rhizome *(tu fu ling)*, Astragalus root *(huang qi)*, Lycium cortex *(di gu pi)*, Moutan root bark *(mu dan pi)*, Red Peony root *(chi shao)*, Licorice root *(gan cao)*

Cogni-Spark™

Typical Applications: Stimulates cognitive functions, post-stroke, vascular dementia, suspected Alzheimer's, Parkinson's, TIA; enhances liver lipotropic functions

Ingredients: 300 mg. Alpha-Glyceryl-Phosphoryl-Choline from soy lecithin

Cold Away™

Typical Applications: Treats colds and flu, fever, sinus, and chest congestion, coughing, aversion to wind, headache, sore throat, tonsillitis, otitis media, measles, pharyngitis

Chinese Therapeutic Actions: Wind-heat, phlegm, cough

Ingredients: Isatis extract leaf and root *(ban lan gen* and *da qing ye)*, Lonicera flower *(jin yin hua)*, Andrographis herb *(chuan xin lian)*, Forsythia fruit *(lian qiao)*, Scute root *(huang qin)*, Platycodon root *(jie geng)*, Wild Chrysanthemum flower *(ye ju hua)*, Citrus peel *(chen pi)*, Angelica root *(bai zhi)*, Magnolia flower *(xin yi hua)*, Xanthium fruit *(cang er zi)*, Licorice root *(gan cao)*

Collagenex™

Typical Applications: Osteoarthritis, rheumatoid arthritis, tendonitis, repair ligaments, connective tissue support

Ingredients: Collagen Type 2 *(Gallus Gallus)*, Grape whole plant extract *(Vitis Vinifera L., Carknooue Cinsault)*

Colostroplex™

Typical Applications: Stops diarrhea, anti-viral, anti-bacterial, anti-fungal

Chinese Therapeutic Actions: Harmonize digestion

Ingredients: Bovine colostrum

Coptis Purge Fire™

Typical Applications: UTI; herpes; intense local inflammation: eye, ear, throat; hives

Chinese Therapeutic Actions: Purge fire and toxins, dry dampness

Ingredients: Coptis rhizome *(huang lian)*, Lophatherum herb *(dan zhu ye)*, Bupleurum root *(chai hu)*, Rehmannia (raw) root *(sheng di huang)*, Tang Kuei root *(dang gui)*, White Peony root *(bai shao)*,

Akebia Trifoliata Caulis *(mu tong),* Anemarrhena root *(zhi mu),* Phellodendron cortex *(huang bai),* Gentiana root *(long dan cao),* Alisma rhizome *(ze xie),* Plantago seed *(che qian zi),* Scute root *(huang qin),* Sophora root *(ku shen),* Forsythia fruit *(lian qiao),* Gardenia fruit *(zhi zi),* Licorice root *(gan cao)*

Cordyceps PS™

Typical Applications: Asthma, wheezing, chronic cough, Chronic Obstructive Pulmonary Disease, pulmonary heart disease, hyperlipidemia, hepatitis, male impotence, chronic fatigue syndrome; strengthen resistance to disease, boost the immune system, and enhance athletic performance

Chinese Therapeutic Actions: Tonify kidney yang, nourish lung yin, strengthen protective qi, stop cough, and transform phlegm

Ingredients: Cordyceps fruiting body (500 mg.) *(dong chong xia cao)*

Coriolus PS™

Typical Applications: Used in conjunction with chemo and radiation therapy, stimulates production of killer T cells and tumor necrosis factor (TNF); activates macrophage function, adjunct for hepatitis, lung infections

Chinese Therapeutic Actions: Dispel dampness, reduce phlegm, clear heat, and alleviate inflammation

Ingredients: Coriolus versicolor *(yun zhi)* extract containing 25% polysaccharides

Drain Dampness™

Typical Applications: Edema, difficulty in urination, sensation of heaviness

Chinese Therapeutic Actions: Stagnation of water and dampness in the body, strengthen the spleen

Ingredients: Alisma rhizome *(ze xie)*, Poria sclerotium *(fu ling)*, Polyporus sclerotium *(zhu ling)*, Cinnamon twig *(gui zhi)*, White Atractylodes rhizome *(bai zhu)*

Ease 2™

Typical Applications: Neck, shoulder, muscle tension; GI disorders, loose stools

Chinese Therapeutic Actions: Invigorate liver qi, harmonize liver/spleen, harmonize exterior/interior, relieve the surface, and tonify spleen qi

Ingredients: Bupleurum root *(chai hu)*, Pueraria root *(ge gen)*, Pinellia rhizome *(ban xia)*, Cinnamon twig *(gui zhi)*, White Peony root *(bai shao)*, Ginseng root *(ren shen)*, Scute root *(huang qin)*, Licorice root *(gan cao)*, Ginger rhizome *(gan jiang)*

Ease Plus™

Typical Applications: Addiction withdrawal, anxiety, insomnia, constipation

Chinese Therapeutic Actions: Invigorate liver qi, sedate liver yang, tonify spleen qi, calm shen

Ingredients: Calcium carbonate *(mu li* and *long gu)*, Bupleurum root *(chai hu)*, Ginseng root *(ren shen)*, Ginger rhizome *(gan jiang)*, Pinellia rhizome *(ban xia)*, Scute root *(huang qin)*, Cinnamon twig *(gui zhi)*, Rhubarb rhizome *(da huang)*, Vladimiria souliei root *(mu xiang)*

Ecliptex™

Typical Applications: Protect and facilitate liver's recovery from disease and toxins, hepatitis

Chinese Therapeutic Actions: Vitalize Qi and blood circulation; tonify kidney, liver yin, and blood

Ingredients: Eclipta herb concentrate *(han lian cao)*, Milk Thistle seed (Silybum) *(silybum marianum)*, Curcuma tuber *(yu jin)*, Salvia root *(dan shen)*, Lycium fruit *(gou qi zi)*, Ligustrum fruit *(nu zhen zi)*, Bupleurum root *(chai hu)*, Schizandra fruit *(wu wei zi)*, Tienchi root *(san qi)*, Tang Kuei root *(dang gui)*, Plantago seed *(che qian zi)*, Licorice root *(gan cao)*

EPAQ™

Typical Applications: Anti-inflammatory activity; nourishes brain function; useful in treatment of hypertension, high triglycerides, diabetes, eczema, psoriasis, lupus, MS, migraine headaches, osteoarthritis, colitis, Crohn's disease, PMS

Ingredients: Neptune Krill oil

Essence Chamber™

Typical Applications: Treats benign prostatic hypertrophy with urinary dysfunction, retention and difficulty of urination, distension and fullness of the lower hypogastrium

Chinese Therapeutic Actions: Clear damp heat from lower burner, clear dampness and promote urination, promote the separation of the Pure and the Turbid in the lower burner, clear the liver channel in the lower burner, circulate stagnant blood, tonify kidney yang

Ingredients: Patrinia herb *(bai jiang cao)*, Saw Palmetto fruit concentrate *(Serenoa repens)*, Salvia root *(dan shen)*, Vaccaria seed *(wang bu liu xing)*, Liquidamber fruit *(lu lu tong)*, Hydrangea fruit (Hydrangae arborscentis), Damiana leaf *(Turnerae aphrodisiacae)*, Poria sclerotium *(fu ling)*, Tokoro rhizome *(bi xie)*, Abutilon seed *(dong kua zi)*

Flavonex™

Typical Applications: Prevent cardiovascular disease; increase cerebral function

Chinese Therapeutic Actions: Dilate peripheral and coronary blood vessels; promote blood circulation; nourish and astringe essence

Ingredients: Pueraria root *(ge gen)*, Ilex root *(mao dong qing)*, Salvia root *(dan shen)*, Lonicera flower *(jin yin hua)*, Eucommia bark *(du zhong)*, Acorus rhizome *(shi chang pu)*, Cistanche salsa herb *(rou cong rong)*, Ho-shou-wu root *(he shou wu)*, Morus fruit *(sang ren)*, Rose fruit *(jin ying zi)*, Lycium fruit *(gou qi zi)*, Zizyphus seed *(suan zao ren)*, Tang Kuei *(dang gui)*, Schizandra fruit *(wu wei zi)*, Ginkgo extract leaf *(yin guo ye)*

Formula H™

Typical Applications: Reduce inflammation of hemorrhoidal tissues, stop hemorrhoidal bleeding, and resolve bloody stools due to other conditions, such as colitis, and Crohn's disease

Chinese Therapeutic Actions: Clear heat and eliminate dampness, consolidate yin, nourish the blood, promote blood circulation, stop bleeding

Ingredients: Sanguisorba root *(di yu)*, Pulsatilla root *(bai tou weng)*, Sophora flower *(huai hua mi)*, White Peony root *(bai shao)*, Tang Kuei root *(dang gui)*, Rehmannia (raw) root *(sheng di huang)*, Fraxinus cortex *(qin pi)*, Phellodendron cortex *(huang bai)*, Lonicera flower *(jin yin hua)*

Formula V™

Typical Applications: Chronic venous insufficiency, varicose veins, pain, heaviness, cramping, itching, swelling of the legs

Ingredients: Horse chestnut seed *(Escin Aesculus hippocastanum)*, Butcher's broom root and rhizome *(Ruscus aculeatus)*, Stoneroot root *(Collinsonia canadensis)*

Ginseng and Gecko™

Typical Applications: Chronic asthma, chronic bronchitis

Chinese Therapeutic Actions: Address lung qi deficiency with heat and yellow/green phlegm; tonify kidney and facilitate the kidney to grasp lung qi

Ingredients: Apricot seed *(ku xing ren)*, Baked Licorice root *(zhi gan cao)*, White Ginseng root *(bai ren shen)*, Poria sclerotium *(fu ling)*, Morus cortex *(sang bai pi)*, Fritillaria bulb *(chuan bei mu)*, Anemarrhena root *(zhi mu)*, Gecko *(ge jie)*

Great Yin™

Typical Applications: Yin deficiency with rising yang; treat night sweats, hot flashes

Chinese Therapeutic Actions: Nourish kidney yin, subdue deficiency fire, clear heat, stop sweating

Ingredients: Rehmannia (cooked) root *(shu di huang)*, Tortoise shell from Chinemys reevesii *(gui ban)*, Phellodendron cortex *(huang bai)*, Anemarrhena root (zhi mu)

Griffonex™ 5-HTP

Typical Applications: Depression, insomnia, headaches, fibromyalgia, PMS, bulimia, weight loss especially to reduce carbohydrate cravings, experimentally used for narcolepsy, seizure disorders

Ingredients: Each capsule contains 50 mg. of L-5-Hydroxytryptophan extracted from Griffonia seeds

Head-Q™

Typical Applications: Headache, neck and shoulder tension

Chinese Therapeutic Actions: Clear exterior wind-cold, move Qi and blood

Ingredients: Magnolia bark *(hou po)*, Chiang-huo rhizome *(qiang huo)*, Angelica root *(bai zhi)*, Ligusticum root *(chuan xiong)*, Siler root *(fang feng)*, Angelica pubescens root *(du huo)*, Vitex fruit *(man jing zi)*, Kao-pen root and rhizome *(gao ben)*, Curcuma tuber *(yu jin)*, Feverfew herb *(Tanacetum parthenium)*

Isatis Cooling™

Typical Applications: Treat Crohn's disease, ulcerative colitis, irritable bowel syndrome, gastric ulcers. Treat hot type leukorrhea accompanied by thick, dark and smelly discharge and abdominal pain. Treat prostate inflammation accompanied by discharge and constant pain, may be used to treat urinary tract infection

Chinese Therapeutic Actions: Clear toxins, clear heat, activate blood circulation

Ingredients: Isatis extract leaf *(da qing ye)*, Isatis extract root *(ban lan gen)*, Codonopsis root *(dang shen)*, Oyster shell *(mu li)*, Bupleurum root *(chai hu)*, Smilax rhizome *(tu fu ling)*, Gardenia fruit *(zhi zi)*, Moutan root bark *(mu dan pi)*, Tang Kuei root *(dang gui)*, Akebia Trifoliata caulis *(mu tong)*, Red Peony root *(chi shao)*, Alisma rhizome *(ze xie)*

Isatis Gold™

Typical Applications: Colds, flu, bronchitis, bacterial and viral infection

Chinese Therapeutic Actions: Clear wind-heat, wind-cold, and phlegm

Ingredients: Isatis extract leaf and root *(ban lan gen* and *da qing ye)*, Echinacea root (Echinacea purpurea), Platycodon root *(jie geng)*, Goldenseal root (Hydrastis canadensis), Ligusticum root *(chuan xiong)*

Licorice 25™

Typical Applications: Viral infections such as viral hepatitis, HIV, inflammatory conditions, canker sores, ulcers, adrenal insufficiency, withdrawal from steroids (prednisone), Chronic Fatigue Syndrome

Chinese Therapeutic Actions: Qi tonic, detoxifier, pain relieving, anti-spasmotic

Ingredients: Licorice root standardized to 25% Glycyrrhizic acid *(gan cao)*

Lily Bulb Formula™

Typical Applications: Dry cough, dry throat, dry nose, bronchitis, pharyngitis, cor pulmonale, tuberculosis, pneumothorax, wheezing, hot palms and soles, night sweats, chronic sore throat

Chinese Therapeutic Actions: Strengthen the lung, nourish yin, stop coughing

Ingredients: Lily bulb *(bai he)*, Rehmannia (raw and cooked) root *(sheng* and *shu di huang)*, Ophiopogon tuber *(mai men dong)*, Fritillaria bulb *(chuan bei mu)*, Platycodon root *(jie geng)*, Tang Kuei root *(dang gui)*, White Peony root *(bai shao)*, Licorice root *(gan cao)*, Scrophularia root *(xuan shen)*

Milk Thistle 80™

Typical Applications: Liver disorders, hepatitis, cirrhosis of the liver, gallstones, psoriasis, and blood sugar imbalance

Ingredients: Milk Thistle (80% Silymarin: *Silybum marianum*); each tablet supplies 160 mg. Silymarin

Mobility 2™

Typical Applications: Arthritis, gout, sciatica, lumbago

Chinese Therapeutic Actions: Relieve the surface, dispel wind-damp, promote the flow of water, and vitalize blood circulation

Ingredients: Red Peony root *(chi shao)*, Tang Kuei root *(dang gui)*, Ligusticum root *(chuan xiong)*, Rehmannia (cooked) root *(shu di huang)*, Persica seed *(tao ren)*, White Atractylodes rhizome *(bai zhu)*, Poria sclerotium *(fu ling)*, Citrus peel *(chen pi)*, Siler root *(fang feng)*, Vitex fruit *(man jing zi)*, Gentiana root *(qin jiao)*, Achyranthes root *(niu xi)*, Chiang-huo rhizome *(qiang huo)*, Clematis root *(wei ling xian)*, Ginger rhizome *(gan jiang)*, Angelica root *(bai zhi)*, Licorice root *(gan cao)*

Nasal Tabs 2™

Typical Applications: Sinusitis, rhinitis, hay fever, colds, flu

Chinese Therapeutic Actions: Release the surface, circulate blood, dispel wind

Ingredients: Xanthium fruit *(cang er zi)*, Cinnamon twig *(gui zhi)*, Red Peony root *(chi shao)*, Ligusticum root *(chuan xiong)*, Angelica root *(bai zhi)*, Cimicifuga rhizome *(sheng ma)*, Licorice root *(gan cao)*, Thyme leaf *(Thymus vulgaris)*, Eucalyptus leaf *(Eucalyptus globulus)*

Nine Flavor Tea™

Typical Applications: Diabetes, sore throat, tidal fever, wasting/thirsting syndrome

Chinese Therapeutic Actions: Nourish liver, kidney, stomach, and spleen yin; clear stomach heat and heart fire; tonify kidney and spleen qi

Ingredients: Rehmannia (raw) root *(sheng di huang)*, Dioscorea root *(shan yao)*, Poria sclerotium *(fu ling)*, Cornus fruit *(shan zhu yu)*, Moutan root bark *(mu dan pi)*, Alisma rhizome *(ze xie)*, Scrophularia root *(xuan shen)*, Glehnia root *(sha shen)*, Ophiopogon tuber *(mai men dong)*

Phellostatin™

Typical Applications: Candidiasis, sinus conditions, cleanse colon, anti-fungal

Chinese Therapeutic Actions: Anti-fungal, tonify spleen and stomach qi

Ingredients: Phellodendron cortex *(huang bai)*, Codonopsis root *(dang shen)*, White Atractylodes rhizome *(bai zhu)*, Anemarrhena root *(zhi mu)*, Plantago seed *(che qian zi)*, Pulsatilla root *(bai tou weng)*, Capillaris herb *(yin chen hao)*, Cnidium fruit *(she chuang zi)*, Houttuynia herb *(yu xing cao)*, Dioscorea root *(shan yao)*, Licorice root *(gan cao)*, Cardamon fruit *(bai dou kou)*

Power Mushrooms™

Typical Applications: Immune enhancement, boost energy

Chinese Therapeutic Actions: Tonify Qi and yin; benefit stomach, spleen, lungs, and kidneys; mildly promote diuresis

Ingredients: Ganoderma (reishi) fruiting body *(ling zhi)*, Tremella fruiting body *(bai mu er)*, Poria sclerotium *(fu ling)*, Polyporus sclerotium *(zhu ling)*

Quercenol

Typical Applications: Prevention of cancer and complications of diabetes, treatment of liver inflammation, anti-aging

Ingredients: Quercetin, Silybum marianum, Proanthocyanidins, Green tea polyphenols, mixed carotenoids, Vitamin E, Vitamin C, Zinc, Selenium

Quiet Digestion™

Typical Applications: Upper/lower gastric distress, travel-related digestive problems

Chinese Therapeutic Actions: Disperse wind and dampness, resolve spleen dampness, regulate the stomach, and resolve phlegm

Ingredients: Poria sclerotium *(fu ling)*, Coix seed *(yi yi ren)*, Shen Chu extract *(shen qu)*, Magnolia bark *(hou po)*, Angelica root *(bai zhi)*, Pueraria root *(ge gen)*, Red Atractylodes rhizome *(cang zhu)*, Vladimiria souliei *(mu xiang)*, Pogostemon herb *(huo xiang)*, Oryza sprout *(gu ya)*, Trichosanthes root *(tian hua fen)*, Chrysanthemum flower *(ju hua)*, Halloysite *(chi shi zhi)*, Red Citrus rind *(ju hong)*, Mentha herb *(bo he)*

Raise Qi™

Typical Applications: Weak limbs, aversion to cold, pale complexion, loose stools, aftermath of severe illness, leukorrhea (cold signs)

Chinese Therapeutic Actions: Tonify Qi, weak pulse, sinking yang

Ingredients: Astragalus root *(huang qi)*, Baked Licorice root *(zhi gan cao)*, Bupleurum root *(chai hu)*, Cimicifuga rhizome *(sheng ma)*, Citrus peel *(chen pi)*, Ginseng root *(ren shen)*, Tang Kuei root *(dang gui)*, White Atractylodes rhizome *(bai zhu)*

Regeneration™

Typical Applications: Enhance the immune system; use as an adjunct to surgery, chemotherapy, and radiation therapy

Chinese Therapeutic Actions: Strengthen the body, clear toxin, stop pain, and harmonize yin and yang

Ingredients: Kirin Ginseng root *(ji lin shen)*, Tang Kuei root *(dang gui)*, Akebia fruit *(ba yue zha)*, Sparganium rhizome *(san leng)*, Zedoaria rhizome *(e zhu)*, Tienchi root *(san qi)*, Gentiana root *(long dan cao)*, Scute root *(huang qin)*, Qin Jiao root *(qin jiao)*, Persica seed *(tao ren)*, Moutan root bark *(mu dan pi)*, White Peony root *(bai shao)*

Rehmannia 8™

Typical Applications: Backache with cold hands/feet, impotence, fatigue

Chinese Therapeutic Actions: Tonify kidney qi and yang, warm the center, benefit the back, and drain dampness

Ingredients: Rehmannia (cooked) herb *(shu di huang)*, Poria sclerotium *(fu ling)*, Moutan root bark *(mu dan pi)*, Dioscorea root *(shan yao)*, Cornus fruit *(shan zhu yu)*, Alisma rhizome *(ze xie)*, Eucommia bark *(du zhong)*, Cinnamon bark *(rou gui)*

Resinall E Tabs™

Typical Applications: Treat pain and swelling due to traumatic injuries (sprains, strains, contusions, fractures, broken bones, torn sinews, bleeding, bruising, lacerations)

Chinese Therapeutic Actions: Promote tissue regeneration, stop bleeding, and activate blood

Ingredients: Enzymes: Bromelain 100 mg., Papain 50 mg., Trypsin 50 mg., Chymotrypsin 100 mcg., Rutin 100 mg.; Herbs: Dragon's Blood resin *(xue jie)*, Tienchi root *(san qi)*, Catechu herb *(er cha)*, Corydalis rhizome *(yan hu suo)*, Carthamus flower *(hong hua)*, Myrrh resin *(mo yao)*, Frankincense gum *(ru xiang)*, Borneol resin *(bing pian)*

Resinall K™

Typical Applications: Pain/swelling from traumatic injury, chronic fixed pain

Chinese Therapeutic Actions: Prevent infections, promote tissue regeneration, stop bleeding, and activate blood

Ingredients: Dragon's blood resin *(xue jie)*, Tienchi root *(san qi)*, Catechu herb *(er cha)*, Corydalis rhizome *(yan hu suo)*, Carthamus *(hong hua)*, Myrrh resin *(mo yao)*, Frankincense gum *(ru xiang)*, Borneol resin *(bing pian)*, alcohol, glycerine

Schizandra Dreams™

Typical Applications: Insomnia, agitation, anxiety attacks

Chinese Therapeutic Actions: Nourish the heart, calm the spirit

Ingredients: Valerian extract *(Valeriana officinalis)*, Oyster shell *(mu li)*, Calcium carbonate *(long gu)*, Schizandra fruit *(wu wei zi)*, Amber resin *(hu po)*, Mandarin essential oil *(Citrus nobilis)*

Shen Gem™

Typical Applications: Insomnia, nervousness, palpitations

Chinese Therapeutic Actions: Vitalize heart blood; tonify spleen, heart qi, and blood; calm shen

Ingredients: Ginseng root *(ren shen)*, Poria sclerotium *(fu ling)*, White Atractylodes rhizome *(bai zhu)*, Zizyphus seed *(suan zao ren)*, Astragalus root *(huang qi)*, Tang Kuei *(dang gui)*, Salvia root *(dan shen)*, Amber resin *(hu po)*, Polygala root *(yuan zhi)*, Longan fruit *(long yan rou)*, Vladimiria Souliei root *(mu xiang)*, Ginger rhizome *(gan jiang)*, Licorice root *(gan cao)*, Cardamon fruit *(sha ren)*

Shen Ling™

Typical Applications: Treat loose stools, diarrhea

Chinese Therapeutic Actions: Tonify spleen and drain dampness

Ingredients: Baked Licorice root *(zhi gan cao)*, Cardamon fruit *(sha ren)*, Citrus peel *(chen pi)*, Codonopsis root *(dang shen)*, Coix seed *(yi yi ren)*, Dioscorea root *(shan yao)*, Dolichos seed *(bai bian dou)*, Lotus seed *(lian zi)*, Platycodon root *(jie geng)*, Poria sclerotium *(fu ling)*, White Atractylodes rhizome *(bai zhu)*

Skin Balance™

Typical Applications: Treat conditions existing in psoriasis, eczema, and other cases of skin inflammation

Chinese Therapeutic Actions: Clear liver heat, eliminate heat and dampness, clean blood

Ingredients: Barbat Skullcap herb *(ban zhi lian)*, Oldenlandia *(bai hua she she cao)*, Gentiana root *(long dan cao)*, Rehmannia (raw) root *(sheng di huang)*, Viola herb *(zi hua di ding)*, Siler root *(fang feng)*, Lonicera flower *(jin yin hua)*, Lysimachia herb *(jin qian cao)*, Coptis rhizome *(huang lian)*, Tang Kuei *(dang gui)*, Bupleurum root *(chai hu)*, Carthamus flower *(hong hua)*, Senna leaf *(fan xie ye)*, Rhubarb rhizome *(da huang)*

Source Qi™

Typical Applications: Cryptosporidiosis, chronic diarrhea with cold signs

Chinese Therapeutic Actions: Strengthen spleen/stomach, tonify Qi, astringe fluids, and increase digestive function

Ingredients: Ailanthus cortex *(chun bai pi)*, Baked Astragalus root *(huang qi)*, White Ginseng root *(bai ren shen)*, White Atractylodes rhizome *(bai zhu)*, Red Atractylodes rhizome *(cang zhu)*, Poria sclerotium *(fu ling)*, Dioscorea root *(shan yao)*, Lotus seed *(lian rou)*, Euryale seed *(qian shi)*, Cimicifuga rhizome *(sheng ma)*, Fried Bupleurum root *(chai hu)*, Charcoaled Ginger *(gan jiang)*, Nutmeg seed *(rou dou kou)*, Baked Licorice root *(zhi gan ao)*, Shen Qu extract *(shen qu)*

SPZM™

Typical Applications: Muscle spasms, particularly due to injury (whiplash) affecting upper body, muscle cramps and restless leg syndrome, neuralgias of the upper body, contractions, numbness in limbs, tremors or lack of strength in limbs, wrist pain carpal tunnel syndrome

Chinese Therapeutic Actions: Invigorate blood, relieve stagnant Qi, moisten and nourish sinews, opens the channels

Ingredients: Calcium aspartate, Clematis root *(wei ling xian)*, Licorice root *(gan cao)*, Magnesium aspartate, Pueraria root *(ge gen)*, Spatholbus root/stem *(ji xue teng)*, White Peony root *(bai shao)*

Stomach Tabs™

Typical Applications: Improves digestion, rids flatulence, relive abdominal bloating and sooths acute and chronic gastritis as well

as gastric and duodenal ulcer, relieves inflammation, help eliminate food allergies, improve absorption of nutrients, motion
sickness

Chinese Therapeutic Actions: Disperse stagnant Qi, disperse food
stagnation, slight warming, resolve spleen dampness and resolve
stomach phlegm

Ingredients: Magnolia bark *(hou po),* Citrus peel *(chen pi),* Pincl-
lia rhizome *(ban xia),* Red Atractylodes rhizome *(cang zhu),* Ginger rhizome *(gan jiang),* Licorice root *(gan cao),* Bupleurum root
(chai hu), Oryza sprout *(gu ya)*

TAMU™

Typical Applications: Eczema, psoriasis, dry skin, skin burns, fungal skin infections, diabetic sores and ulcers, acne, anal fissures,
hives, bedsores, chapped feet and hands, insect bites, diaper rash.
Nerve, muscle and joint pain especially of hot type such as sin-
gles, sciatica, bursitis, post herpetic neuralgia, tendonitis

Ingredients: Tamanu oil *(Calophllum inophyllum),* Avocado oil,
Peppermint essential oil

Unlocking™

Typical Applications: Addresses menstrual pain with heat signs,
endometriosis, ovarian cysts, uterine fibroids, chronic PID, chronic
abnormal vaginal discharge and various stages of cervical intraep-
ithelial neoplasia (cervical dysplasia) with heat signs

Chinese Therapeutic Actions: Clear bound Qi, stagnant Qi and
stasis of blood, clear heat and dampness in lower jiao

Ingredients: Cimicifuga rhizome *(sheng ma)*, Citrus fruit *(zhi ke)*, Cyathula root *(chuan niu xi)*, Fennel fruit *(xiao hui xiang)*, Melia fruit *(chuan lian zi)*, Moutan root bark *(mu dan pi)*, Patrinia herb *(bai jiang cao)*, Phellodendron cortex *(huang bai)*, Poria sclerotium *(fu ling)*, Red Atractylodes rhizome *(cang zhu)*, Red Peony root *(chi shao)*, Sargentodoxa herb *(da xue teng)*, White Atractylodes rhizome *(bai zhu)*

Vinpurazine™

Typical Applications: Cerebral circulation, may improve memory, protects nerve cells, helps in post-stroke and seizure recovery

Ingredients: Rosemary leaf extract, Club Moss extract from Huperzia serrata, Vinpocetine from Vinca minor

Woman's Balance™

Typical Applications: PMS with abdominal bloating and breast swelling, menstrual irregularity, menopausal distress, mild cramps, relieves depression, usefule I treating hepatitis and liver cirrhosis, liver fire headaches, IBS

Chinese Therapeutic Actions: Invigorate congested liver qi, nourish liver blood and yin, strengthen spleen qi, and harmonize liver and spleen

Ingredients: Bupleurum root *(chai hu)*, Citrus peel *(chen pi)*, Cyperus rhizome *(xiang fu)*, Gardenia fruit *(zhi zi)*, Ginger rhizome *(gan jiang)*, Licorice root *(gan cao)*, Moutan root bark *(mu dan pi)*, Poria sclerotium *(fu ling)*, Salvia root *(dan shen)*, Tang Kuei root *(dang gui)*, White Atractylodes rhizome *(bai zhu)*, White Peony root *(bai shao)*

Xanthium Relieve Surface™

Typical Applications: Sinus allergies, poison oak, itching

Chinese Therapeutic Actions: Clear surface wind-heat, open nasal passages, cool heat and dispel wind-dampness, remove toxins

Ingredients: Xanthium fruit *(cang er zi)*, Magnolia flower *(xin yi hua)*, Platycodon root *(jie geng)*, Schizandra fruit *(wu wei zi)*, Angelica root *(bai zhi)*, Wild Chrysanthemum flower *(ye ju hua)*, Siler root *(fang feng)*, Schizonepeta herb *(jing jie)*, Astragalus root *(huang qi)*, White Atractylodes root *(bai zhu)*, Licorice root *(gan cao)*

Yin Chao Jin™

Typical Applications: Cold, flu, sore throat

Chinese Therapeutic Actions: Disperse wind-heat, clear heat and relieve toxins, diaphoretic

Ingredients: Lonicera flower *(jin yin hua)*, Forsythia fruit *(lian qiao)*, Isatis extract root and leaf *(ban lan gen* and *da qing ye)*, Arctium fruit *(niu bang zi)*, Mentha herb *(bo he)*, Schizonepeta herb *(jing jie)*, Soja sprout *(dan dou chi)*, Platycodon root *(jie geng)*, Lophatherum herb *(dan zhu ye)*, Phragmites rhizome *(lu gen)*, Licorice root *(gan cao)*

Yin Chao Junior™

Typical Applications: Colds, fever, coughing, vomiting, and diarrhea in children

Chinese Therapeutic Actions: Clear heat, harmonize digestion, moisten throat and lung, and invigorate blood

Ingredients: Forsythia flower *(lian qiao)*, Morus leaf *(sang ye)*, Shen Qu herb *(shen qu)*, Ephemerantha Fimbriata herb *(you gua shi hu)*, Glehnia stem *(sha shen)*, Fritillaria bulb *(zhe bei mu)*, Platycodon root *(jie geng)*, Eriobotrya leaf *(pi pa ye)*, Microcos paniculata leaf *(po bu ye)*, Pu Er Tea *(pu er cha)*, Trichosanthes peel *(gua lou pi)*, Pinellia tuber *(ban xia)*, Chrysanthemum flower *(ju hua)*, Mentha herb *(bo he)*, Peucedanum root *(qian hu)*, Aurantium fruit *(zhi shi)*, Gardenia fruit *(zhi zi)*, Eupatorium herb *(pei lan)*, Perilla leaf *(zi su ye)*, alcohol, glycerine

Zaocys

Typical Applications: Itching due to allergy, eczema or psoriasis, arthritis with hot joints

Chinese Therapeutic Actions: Dispel wind and dampness, calm internal wind

Ingredients: Zaocys *(wu shao she)*, Tribulus *(bai ji li)*, Cicada *(chan tui)*, Red Peony *(chi shao)*, Tang Kuei *(dang gui)*, Schizonepeta *(jing jie)*, Siler *(fang feng)*, Cnidium *(she chuang zi)*, Licorice *(gan cao)*

Common Acupuncture Points Used in the Treatment of Immune Disorders

Manipulation of acupuncture points either through needling or acupressure can be very effective in treating immune disorders. Practitioners may find the following guide helpful in selecting suitable points.

Symptom(s)	Points
Anxiety	M-HN-3 *(yin tang)*, P-6, P-5 *(jian shi)*, H-7 *(shen men)*, S-36 *(zu san li)*, P-7 *(da ling)*, Gv-24 *(shen ting)*, H-5 *(tong li)*, H-6 *(yin xi)*, Gv-19 *(hou ding)*, B-15 *(xin shu)*, Co-14 *(ju que)*, Gv-19 *(hou ding)*, B-15 *(xin shu)* Ear points: shen men, heart, subcortex, sympathetic

Symptom(s)	Points
Cough	Gv-14 *(da zhui)*, Gv-12 *(shen zhu)*, Gv-10 *(ling tai)*, B-13 *(fei shu)*, L-5 *(chi ze)*, L-7 *(lie que)*, L-10 *(yu ji)*, LI-4 *(he gu)*, LI-11 *(qu chi)*, SJ-5 *(wai guan)*, L-5 *(chi ze)*, L-1 *(zhong fu)*, S-40 *(feng long)*, Gv-14 *(da zhui)*, Gv-12 *(shen zhu)*, Gv-10 *(ling tai)*, L-6 *(kong zui)*, Co-17 *(shan zhong)*, SJ-6 *(zhi gou)*, P-7 *(da ling)*, L-1 *(zhong fu)*, Co-17 *(shan zhong)*, B-13 *(fei shu)*, Gv-14 *(da zhui)*, L-9 *(tai yuan)*
Depression (sadness)	P-6 *(nei guan)*, S-36 *(zu san li)*, L-3 *(tai chong)*, L-4 *(four gates)*, Sp-6 *(san yin jiao)*, B-20 *(pi shu)*, Gv-20 *(bai hui)*, Co-6 *(qi hai)* Ear: depression, shen men
Dizziness	GB-20 *(feng chi)*, B-18 *(gan shu)*, Li-3 *(tai chong)*, GB-43 *(xia xi)*, P-6 *(nei guan)*, GB-34 *(yang ling quan)*, ah shi points on upper back neckB-23 *(shen shu)*, K-3 *(tai xi)*, Sp-6 *(san yin jiao)*, Li-3 *(tai chong)*, B-15 *(xin shu)*, K-1 *(yong quan)*, P-6 *(nei guan)*, GB-2 *(ting hui)*
Fatigue	Gv-20 *(bai hu)*, B-62 *(shen mai)*, Sp-6 *(san yin jiao)*, Co-12 *(zhong wan)*, S-36 *(zu san li)*, GB-20 *(feng chi)*, Co-6 *(qi hai)*, K-3 *(tai xi)*, Li-3 *(tai chong)*, K-6 *(zhao hai)*, Sp-3 *(tai bai)*, B-20 *(pi shu)*, M-HN-1 *(si shen cong)*, B-52 *(fu xi)*, B-23 *(shen shu)*, Gv-4 *(ming men)*, H-3 *(shao hai)*, H-7 *(shen men)*, B-15 *(xin shu)*, B-17 *(ge shu)*, M-HN-3 *(yin tang)*, Co-4 *(guan yuan)*, P-6 *(nei guan)*
Fever	P-3 *(qu ze)*, B-40 *(yi xi)*, B-54 *(wei zhong)*, P-9 *(zong chong)*, Gv-26 *(ren zhong)*, Gv-14 *(da zhui)*, LI-11 *(qu chi)*, LI-4 *(he gu)*, S-44 *(nei ting)*, S-37 *(shang ju xu)*, S-25 *(tian shu)*, N-CA-3 *(zhi xie)*, Li-3 *(tai chong)*

Symptom(s)	Points
General health support	Li-3 *(tai chong)*, Sp-6 *(san yin jiao)*, S-36 *(zu san li)*, Li-11 *(yin lian)*, self-massage thymus area
Impotence	Gv-20 *(bai hui)*, Co-12 *(zhong wan)*, Co-6 *(qi hai)*, Co-4 *(guan yuan)*, B-23 *(shen shu)*, B-30 *(bai huang shu)*, K-3 *(tai xi)*, Gv-4 *(ming men)*
Insomnia	P-6 *(nei guan)*, P-7 *(da ding)*, K-3 *(tai xi)*, H-7 *(shen men)*, H-8 *(shao fu)*, Gv-20 *(bai hui)*, L-7 *(lie que)*, Sp-6 *(san yin jiao)*, L-7 *(lie que)*, K-3 *(tai xi)*, H-7 *(shen men)*, M-HN-3 *(yin tang)*, N-HN-5 *(zeng ming)*
Jaundice	Gv-9 *(zhi yang)*, SI-4 *(wan gu)*, B-19 *(dan shu)*, GB-34 *(yang ling quan)*, Sp-9 *(yin ling quan)*, Li-3 *(tai chong)*, P-6 *(nei guan)*, Li-14 *(qi men)*, SJ-6 *(zhi gou)*, Li-13 *(zhang men)*
Lymph drainage (phlegm herbs)	S-40 *(feng long)*, Sp-3 *(tai bai)*, SI-3 *(hou xi)*, B-62 *(shen mai)*, GB-20 *(feng chi)*, Gv-14 *(da zhui)*, Gv-8 *(jin suo)*, Gv-16 *(feng fu)*, B-20 *(pi shu)*, Gv-20 *(bai hu)*, B-23 *(shen shu)*, GB-34 *(yang ling quan)*, Sp-6 *(san yin jiao)*, S-36 *(zu san li)*, Co-12 *(zhong wan)*, S-8 *(tou wei)*, Co-12 *(zhong wan)*, Sp-5 *(shang qiu)*, P-6 *(nei guan)*, P-5 *(jian shi)*, GB-40 *(qiu xu)*, S-40 *(feng long)*, S-41 *(jie xi)*
Nasal congestion	L-7 *(lie que)*, LI-4 *(he gu)*, LI-11 *(qu chi)*, M-HN-3 *(yin tang)*, LI-20 *(ying xiang)*, Gv-23 *(shang xing)*, B-2 *(zan zhu)*, M-HN-14 *(bi tong)*, M-HN-9 *(tai yang)*, SJ-5 *(wai guan)*, GB-20 *(feng chi)*, Li-2 *(xing jian)*, Li-3 *(tai chong)*, GB-39 *(xuan zhong)*, Gv-23 *(shang xing)*, LI-20 *(ying xiang)*

Symptom(s)	Points
Pain	B-60 *(kun lun)*, B-58 *(fei yang)*, B-59 *(fu yang)*, B-36 *(fu fen)*, B-37 *(po hu)*, GB-30 *(huan tiao)*, GB-31 *(feng shi)*, GB-34 *(yang ling quan)*, GB-39 *(xuan zhong)*, SI-3 *(hou xi)*, B-62 *(shen mai)*, LI-4 *(he gu)*, P-6 *(nei guan)*, B-23 *(shen shu)*, B-25 *(da chang shu)*, B-54 *(wei zhong)*, B-28 *(pang guang shu)*, M-BW-25 *(shi qi zhui xia)*, L1-L5 *(Hua tuo jia ji)* points if tender
Urination Difficulty	GB-41 *(zu ling qi)*, SJ-5 *(wai guan)*, Co-3 *(zhong ji)*, Sp-6 *(san yin jiao)*, Sp-9 *(yin ling quan)*, K-6 *(zhao hai)*, B-28 *(pang guang shu)*, B-22 *(san jiao shu)*, K-7 *(fu liu)*, S-28 *(shui dao)*, L-7 *(lie que)*, B-13 *(fei shu)*, Co-3 *(zhong ji)*, Co-9 *(shui fen)*, P-6 *(nei guan)*, GB-34 *(yang ling quan)*
Urination Frequency/ Incontinence	B-23 *(shen shu)*, Co-4 *(guan yuan)*, Sp-6 *(san yin jiao)*, K-2 *(ran gu)*, B-53 *(wei yang)*, K-3 *(tai xi)*, K-6 *(zhao hai)*, Co-4 *(guan yuan)*, K-3 *(tai xi)*, Sp-6 *(san yin jiao)*, SI-3 *(hou xi)*, Gv-26 *(ren zhong)*, K-11 *(heng gu)*
Wind-Cold	GB-20 *(feng chi)*, B-12 *(feng men)*, B-13 *(fei shu)*, L-7 *(lie qu)*, LI-4 *(he gu)*
Wind-Heat	Co-22 *(tian tu)*, SJ-6 *(zhi gou)*, LI-4 *(he gu)*, LI-18 *(fu tu)*, L-6 *(kong zui)*, L-10 *(yu ji)*, LI-11 *(qu chi)*, M-HN-30 *(bai lao)*, L-11 *(shao shang)*, SI-17 *(tian rong)*

Resources

For further information, a list of practitioners in your area who recommend herbs, and/or information about seminars or our upcoming newsletter, write to the author:

Andrew Gaeddert
c/o Get Well Foundation
8001A Capwell Drive
Oakland, CA 94621
Phone: 510-635-9778
Fax: 510-639-9140
E-mail: info@GetWellFoundation.org

The following organization helps protect the freedom of Americans to use vitamins and herbal products:

Citizens for Health
2104 Stevens Avenue South
Minneapolis, MN 55404
Phone: 612-879-7585
Website: www.citizens.org

The following organizations or agencies that offer information and support to persons with immune disorders.

AIDS.ORG
7985 Santa Monica Boulevard, #99
West Hollywood, CA 90046
Phone: CDC National AIDS Hotline: (800) 342-2437
Website: www.aids.org

ALS Association, National Office
27001 Agoura Road, Suite 150
Calabasas Hills, CA 91301-5104
Phone: 818-880-9007
Fax: 818-880-9006
Website: www.alsa.org

American Apitherapy Society
5535 Balboa Bl., Suite 225
Encino, CA 91316
Phone: 818-501-0446
Fax 818-995-9334
Website: www.apitherapy.org

American Autoimmune Related Diseases Association
National Office
22100 Gratiot Avenue
East Detroit, MI 48021
Phone: (586) 776-3900
E-mail: aarda@aol.com
Website: www.aarda.org

American Cancer Society
Phone: 1-800-227-2345
TTY: 1-866-228-4327

The American Lung Association
61 Broadway, 6th Floor
NY, NY 10006
Phone: 1-800-586-4872
Phone: 212-315-8700
Website: www.lungusa.org

American Sleep Apnea Association
1424 K Street NW, Suite 302
Washington, DC 20005
Phone: 202-293-3650
Fax: 202-293-3656
Website: www.sleepapnea.org

American Thyroid Association
Phone: 1-800-849-7643
Website: www.thyroid.org

Arthritis Foundation
P.O. Box 7669
Atlanta, GA 30357-0669
Phone: 1-800-568-4045
Website: www.arthritis.org

The CFIDS Association of America
P.O. Box 220398
Charlotte, NC 28222-0398
Phone: 704-365-2343
Website: www.cfids.org

Crohn's and Colitis Foundation of America (CCFA), Inc., National Headquarters
386 Park Avenue South, 17th Floor
New York, NY 10016-8804
Phone: 212-685-3440
Phone: 1-800-932-2423
Fax: 212-779-4098
E-mail: info@ccfa.org
Website: www.ccfa.org

Guillain-Barré Syndrome Foundation International
P.O. Box 262
Wynnewood, PA 19096
Phone: 610-667-0131
Fax: 610-667-7036
E-mail: info@gbsfi.com
Website: www.gbsfi.com

International Scleroderma Network
7455 France Avenue So., #266
Edina, MN 55435 USA
Phone: 1-800-564-7099
Website: www.sclero.org

Lupus Foundation of America, Inc.
2000 L Street NW, Suite 710
Washington, DC 20036
Phone: 202-349-1155 or 800-558-0121
Phone: Health Educator: 202-349-1159

Lyme Disease Association, Inc.
P.O. Box 1438
Jackson, NJ 08527
Phone: 888-366-6611
Fax: 732 938-7215
E-mail: LYMELITER@aol.com
Website: www.LymeDiseaseAssociation.org

Myasthenia Gravis Foundation of America
1821 University Avenue W., Suite S256
St. Paul, MN 55104
Phone: 651-917-6256 or 1-800-541-5454
Fax: 651-917-1835
E-mail: mgfa@myasthenia.org
Website: www.myasthenia.org

National Adrenal Diseases Foundation
505 Northern Boulevard, Suite 200
Great Neck, NY 11021
Phone: 516-487-4992
E-mail: nadfmail@aol.com
Website: www.medhelp.org/nadf/

National Headache Foundation
820 N. Orleans, Suite 217
Chicago, IL 60610
Phone: 1-888-643-5552
Website: www.headaches.org

National Institute of Diabetes and Digestive and Kidney Diseases
Office of Communications and Public Liaison
NIDDK, NIH
Building 31, Room 9A04
31 Center Drive
MSC 2560
Bethesda, MD 20892-2560
E-mail: dkwebmaster@extra.niddk.nih.gov
Website: www.niddk.nih.gov/

National Meniere's Disease Foundation, Inc.
335 Main Street
Red Hill PA 18076
Phone: 215-541-1473
Website: www.homestead.com/NMDF

The National Multiple Sclerosis Society
733 Third Avenue
New York, NY 10017
Phone: 1-800-344-4867
Website: www.nationalmssociety.org

National Organization for Rare Disorders
55 Kenosia Avenue
P.O. Box 1968
Danbury, CT 06813-1968
Phone: 203-744-0100
TDD: 203-797-9590
Fax: 203-798-2291
Website: www.rarediseases.org

National Psoriasis Foundation
6600 SW 92nd Avenue, Suite 300
Portland, OR 97223-7195
Phone: 503-244-7404 or 800-723-9166
Fax: 503-245-0626
E-mail: getinfo@psoriasis.org
Website: www.psoriasis.org

The Neuropathy Association, Inc.
P.O. Box 26226
New York, NY 10117-3422
Phone: 212-692-0662
Website: www.neuropathy.org

Reiter's Information & Support Group Inc.
1105 D 15th Avenue, #172
Longview, WA 98632-3068
Phone: 360-423-9374 or 877-800-7474
Website: www.risg.org

Sjögren's Syndrome Foundation
8120 Woodmont Avenue, Suite 530
Bethesda, MD 20814
Phone: 301-718-0300
Fax: 301-718-0322
Website: www.sjogrens.org

Spondylitis Association of America
P.O. Box 5872
Sherman Oaks, CA 91413
Phone: 1-800-777-8189 or 1-818-981-1616
E-mail: info@spondylitis.org
Website: www.spondylitis.org

Bibliography

Andreas, Steve, and Faulker, Charles, eds., *NLP: The New Technology of Achievement* (New York, NY: William Morrow and Company, 1994).

APUA Newsletter 19(2) (2001),

Batmanghelidj, F., "A New and Natural Method of Treatment of Peptic Ulcer Disease," *Journal of Clinical Gastroenterology* 5 (1983): 203–205.

Batmanghelidj, F., *Your Body's Many Cries for Water* (Falls Church, VA: Global Health Solutions).

Bensky, Dan, Clavey, Steven, and Stöger, Erich, with Andrew Gamble, *Chinese Herbal Medicine: Materia Medica*

Berkow, Robert, M.D., ed., *Merck Manual of Medical Information, Home Edition* (Pocket Books, 1997).

Brechka, Nicole, "Living with Lupus," *Let's Live* (October 2001), 60.

Brekman II, and Dardymov IV, "New substances of plan origin which increase nonspecific resistance," *Ann. Rev. Pharm.* (1969), 9:419–30.

Breneman, J. C., *Basics of Food Allergy* (Springfield, IL: Charles C. Thomas, 1978).

Budd, Martin, M.D., *Low Blood Sugar* (New York, NY: Sterling Publishing, 1981).

Buffington, C. "Vitamin D Deficiency in the Morbidly Obese," *Obes Surg* (1993), 3(4), 421–24.

Carper, Jean, "Eat Smart," *USA Weekend* (Nov. 16–18, 2001), 6.

Carper, Jean, *Food:Your Miracle Medicine* (New York: HarperCollins, 1993), 43.

Carter, Joseph J. "Liver Protection and Repair: Synthesizing Herbal Science and Chinese Energetics," *Health Concerns Professional Newsletter* 3(1)4.

Cascinu, S., et al., "Neuroprotective Effect of Reduced Glutathione on Oxaliplatin-Based Chemotherapy in Advanced Colorectal Cancer: A Randomized, Double-Blind, Placebo-Controlled Trial," *Journal of Clinical Oncology* 20 (2002), 3478–83.

Challem, Jack, "How to Save Your Skin," *Let's Live* (April 1999), 43.

Challem, Jack, *The Inflammation Syndrome* (Hoboken, NJ: John Wiley & Sons, Inc., 2003).

Chang, Hson-Mou, Ph.D., and But, Paul Pui-Hay, Ph.D., eds., *Pharmacology and Applications of Chinese Materia Medica* (World Scientific Publishing Co. Pte. Ltd., 1986, 1987).

Chu, D. T., et al., "Astragalus Root," *American Herbal Pharmacopoeia and Therapeutic Compendium* (Aug. 1999).

Citizens for Health Report 2(1) (1994).

Clark, L. C., et al., "Effects of Selenium Supplementation for Cancer Prevention in Patients with Carcinoma of the Skin," *JAMA* 276 (1996), 1957–63.

Colt, H. G., and Shapiro, A. G., "Drug-Induced Illness as a Cause for Admission to a Community Hospital." *Journal of the American Geriatrics Society* Vol. 37 (1989), 323–26.

Fawzi, Wafaie W.; Hunter, David J.; Kupka, Roland; Morris, Steve; Mugusi, Ferdinand; Msamanga, Gernard I.; and Spiegelman, Donna, "Selenium Status Is Associated with Accelerated HIV Disease Progression among HIV-1-Infected Pregnant Women in Tanzania," *J. Nutr* 134 (2004), 2556–60.

Fawzy, F. I., et al., "Malignant Melanoma. Effects of an Early Structured Psychiatric Intervention, Coping, and Affective State on Recurrence and Survival 6 Years Later," *Arch Gen Psychiatry* 50(9) (September 1993), 681–89.

Foster, Steven, and Chongxi, Yue, *Herbal Emissaries: Bringing Chinese Herbs to the West: A Guide to Gardening, Herbal Wisdom, and Well-Being* (Rochester, VT: Healing Arts Press, 1992).

Fuchs, Nan Kathryn, *Modified Citrus Pectin (MCP): A Super Nutraceutica* (North Bergen, NJ: Basic Health Publications, 2003).

Gaeddert, Andrew, *Healing Digestive Disorders, Second Edition* (Berkeley, CA: North Atlantic Books, 1998, 2004).

Goldberg, Alice, and Brinckmann, Josef, eds., *Herbal Medicine* (Integrative Medicine Communications, 2000).

Grant, W. B., "An Estimate of Premature Cancer Mortality in the U.S. Due to Inadequate Doses of Solar Ultraviolet-B Radiation," *Cancer* 94(6) (2002), 1867–75.

Holt, Stephen, M.D., and Comac, Linda. *Miracle Herbs: How Herbs Combine with Modern Medicine to Treat Cancer, Heart Disease, AIDS, and More* (Carol Publishing Group, 1998).

Hu, Y-J, et al., "The Protective Role of Selenium on the Toxicity of Cisplatin-Contained Chemotherapy Regimen in Cancer Patients," *Biol Trace Elem Res* 56 (1997), 331–41.

Huisman, A. M., et al., "Vitamin D Levels in Women with Systemic Lupus Erythematosis and Fibromyalgia," *J. Rheumatol* 28(11) (2001), 2535–39.

Jedrychowski, W., et al., "Nutrient Intake Patterns in Gastric and Colorectal Cancers," *Int J Occup Med Environ Health* 14(4) (2001), 391–95.

Jinhuang, Zhou, et al., eds., "Recent Advances in Chinese Herbal Drugs," *Science Press* 14 and *S.A.T.A.S.* (1991), 141–47.

Journal of General Internal Medicine (Jan. 2005 issue).

Kabat-Zinn, Jon, *Wherever You Go, There You Are* (New York, NY: St. Martin's Press, 1994).

Kolata, Gina, "Questions Grow Over Usefulness of Some Routine Cancer Tests," *New York Times* CLI(51) (December 30, 2001), 983, www.nytimes.com.

Kupin, V., "Reishi Mushroom: Ganoderma Lucidum," *American Herbal Pharmacopoeia and Therapeutic Compendium* (Sept. 2000), 14.

Liebgold, Howard, M.D., *Curing Anxiety, Phobias, Shyness and OCD, the Phobease Way* (Angelnet, 2001), 78–79.

Liu, G. T., "Pharmacological Actions and Clinical Uses of Fructus Schizandrae." In Zhou, J., Liu, G. T., Chen J., editor(s), *Recent Advances in Chinese Herbal Drugs—Actions and Uses* (Beijing: Science Press, 1991), p. 100–11.

Mahon, B. D., et al., "Cytokine Profile in Patients with Multiple Sclerosis Following Vitamin D Supplementation," *J Neuoimmunol* 134(1–2) (2003), 128–32.

Mayne, S. T., et. al., "Nutrient intake and risk of subtypes of esophageal and gastric cancer." *Cancer Epidemiol. Biomarkers Prev.,* 10:1055–62, 2001

McCaleb, Robert, et al., *The Encyclopedia of Popular Herbs: From the Herb Research Foundation, Your Complete Guide to the Leading Medicinal Plants* (Prima Lifestyles, 2000).

Mills, Simon, and Boone, Kerry, *Principles and Practice of Phytotherapy: Modern Herbal Medicine* (Harcourt Publishers Ltd., 2000).

Morazzoni, P., and Bombardelli, F., "Astragalus Root," *American Herbal Pharmacopoeia and Therapeutic Compendium* (Aug. 1999), 15.

Murray, Michael T. *The Healing Power of Herbs: The Enlightened Person's Guide to the Wonders of Medicinal Plants, Second Edition* (Prima Publishing, 1992, 1995).

Ni, Maoshing, *Yellow Emperor's Classic of Medicine: A New Translation in the Neijing Suwen with Commentary* (Shambhala, 1995).

Pizzorno, Joseph E., Jr., and Murray, Michael T., eds., *Textbook of Natural Medicine, Second Edition* (Churchill Livingstone, 1993, 1999).

Scannell, Kate, M.D., "Medical Marijuana," *San Francisco Chronicle* (Feb. 16, 2003), D3.

Sheldon, Saul, et al., eds., *PDR for Nutritional Supplements* (Medical Economics Company, Inc., 2001).

Slattery, M. L., et al., "Carotenoids and Colon Cancer," *American Journal of Clinical Nutrition* 71(2) (Feb. 2000), 575–82.

Spiegel, David, M.D., *Living Beyond Limits: New Hope & Help for Facing Life-Threatening Illness* (New York: Times Books, 1993).

Sternbach, Richard, *Mastering Pain: A Twelve Step Program for Coping with Chronic Pain* (Ballantine Books, 1988).

Subhuti Dharmandada, *Chinese Herbal Therapies for Immune Disorders* (Institute for Traditional Medicine and Preventative Health Care, 1988).

Suzuki, F., Kobayashi, M., Komatsu, Y., Kato, A., and Pollard, R. B. "*Keishi-ka-kei-to,* A Traditional Chinese Herbal Medicine Inhibits Pulmonary Metastasis of $B_{16,}$ Melanoma," *Anticancer Res* 17 (1997), 873–78.

Terry, P., et al., "Dietary Intake of Folic Acid and Colorectal Cancer Risk in a Cohort of Women," *Int J Cancer* 97(6) (Feb. 20, 2002), 864–67.

Thondup, Tulka, *The Healing Power of Mind* (Shambhala Publications, Inc., 1996).

Toniolo, P., et al., "Serum Carotenoids and Breast Cancer," *Am J Epidemiol* 153(12) (June 15, 2001), 1142–47.

Vasquez, D.C., N.D., Alex, Manso, M.D., Gilbert, Cannell, M.D., John, "The Clinical Importance of Vitamin D (Cholecalerferol): A Paradigm Shift with Implications for All Health Care Providers," *Alternative Therapies in Health and Medicine* 10(5) (Sept./Oct. 2004).

Yance, Donald, and Valentine, Arlene, *Herbal Medicine, Healing & Cancer, First Edition* (McGraw-Hill, 1999).

Zhang, Y. D., Shen, J. P., Zhu, S. H., Huang, D. K., Ding, Y., Zhang, X. L. "Effects of astragalus (ASI, SK) on experimental liver injury. *Yaoxue Yuebao* 27(6): 401–6.

Zhu-Fan, Xie, *Best of Traditional Chinese Medicine* (New World Press, 1995).

Website References

ALS Association, www.alsa.org/.

American Autoimmune Related Diseases Association, www.aarda.org.

American Botanical Council, "Immunomodulating Compounds from Traditional Chinese Herbs," www.herbalgram.org.

Arthritis.com, www.arthritis.com/nsaids.asp. Accessed October 2, 2004.

Crayhon, Robert, "The Paleolithic Diet and Its Modern Implications: An Interview with Loren Cordain, Ph.D.," www.chetday.com/cordaininterview.htm.

Emerson Ecologics, *Preventing Childhood Leukemia with Folic Acid,* www.emersonecologics.com.

Five Questions You Should Ask, If You Have Cancer, www.wsj.com.

Harvard School of Public Health, "Risk of Lung Cancer May Be Reduced by Eating a Wide Variety of Fruits and Vegetables," http://www.hsph.harvard.edu/press/releases/press10122000b.html.

Kirchheimer, Sid, "Soy Improves Prostate Cancer Outlook," http://my.webmd.com/content/article/94/102884.htm?z=3734_00000_1000_ts_02.

Mayo Clinic Staff, "Chickenpox" (September 23, 2004), www.MayoClinic.com.

Mayo Clinic Staff, "NSAIDs: How to Avoid Side Effects," www.mayoclinic.com/invoke.cfm?objectid=E08D9F67-76D9-4D8F-B953CCEF9693D005. Accessed October 2, 2004.

National Cancer Institute, "Antioxidants and Cancer Prevention," www.cancer.gov/cancertopics/factsheet/antioxidantsprevention.

National Institute of Mental Health, "Antidepressant Medications," www.mental-health-matters.com/articles/nimh001.php?artID=236#ptdep7. Accessed October 5, 2004.

National Institute of Neurological Disorders and Stroke, "NINDS Guillain-Barre Syndrome Information Page," www.ninds.nih.gov/disorders/gbs/gbs.htm.

National Library of Medicine, "Allergic Rhinitis," www.nlm.nih.gov/medlineplus/ency/article/000813.htm. Accessed October 1, 2004.

National Women's Health Information Center, "Thyroid Disorders," www.4woman.gov/faq/thyroid_disease.htm. Accessed October 6, 2004.

NIDDK Office of Health Research Reports, "Addison's
Disease: Adrenal Insufficiency," NIH Publication No. 04-3054
(June 2004), www.niddk.nih.gov/health/endo/pubs/addison/
addison.htm.

Nordenberg, Tamar, "Tossing and Turning No More: How to
Get a Good Night's Sleep," *FDA Consumer* (July–August
1998), www.fda.gov/fdac/features/1998/498_sleep.html.

Nutritional Outlook, www.nutritionaloutlook.com.

PlanetHerbs Online, www.planetherbs.com.

U.C. Davis Health System, "Breast Cancer,"
www.ucdmc.ucdavis.edu/healthconsumers/health/
000006.shtml.

U.S. Department of Health and Human Services, "Over-the-
Counter Drugs Aren't Risk Free," www.healthfinder.gov.
Accessed October 2, 2004.

WebMD Inc., www.WebMD.com.

WholeHealthMD.com, "NAC (N-acetylcysteine),"
www.wholehealthmd.com/refshelf/substances_view/
1,1525,809,00.html.

Notes

Chapter One

1. American Autoimmune Related Diseases Association, www.aarda.org.
2. Ni, Maoshing, *Yellow Emperor's Classic of Medicine; A New Translation of the Neijing Suwen with Commentary* (Shambhala), 1995.
3. Zhu-Fan, Xie, *Best of Traditional Chinese Medicine* (New World Press, 1995), 28.
4. Pizzorno, Joseph E., Jr., and Murray, Michael T., eds., *Textbook of Natural Medicine, Second Edition* (Churchill Livingstone, 1993, 1999), 321.
5. Pizzorno and Murray, 323.
6. Liebgold, Howard, M.D., *Curing Anxiety, Phobias, Shyness and OCD, the Phobease Way* (Angelnet 2001), 78–79.
7. Thondup, Tulka, *The Healing Power of Mind* (Shambhala Publications, Inc., 1996), 65.
8. Spiegel, David, M.D., *Living Beyond Limits: New Hope & Help for Facing Life-Threatening Illness* (New York: Times Books, 1993), 77.

9. Fawzy, F. I., et al., "Malignant Melanoma. Effects of an Early Structured Psychiatric Intervention, Coping, and Affective State on Recurrence and Survival 6 Years Later," *Arch Gen Psychiatry* 50(9) (September 1993), 681–89.
10. Spiegel, 88.
11. www.planetherbs.com.
12. National Women's Health Information Center, "Thyroid Disorders," www.4woman.gov/faq/thyroid_disease.htm. Accessed October 6, 2004.
13. Thondup, 33.
14. "Five Questions You Should Ask, If You Have Cancer," www.wsj.com.
15. Andreas, Steve, and Faulker, Charles, eds., *NLP: The New Technology of Achievement* (New York, NY: William Morrow and Company, 1994), 56.
16. Kabat-Zinn, Jon, *Wherever You Go, There You Are* (New York, NY: St. Martin's Press, 1994).
17. Adapted from: Sternbach, Richard, *Mastering Pain: A Twelve Step Program for Coping with Chronic Pain* (Ballantine Books, 1988).
18. Words and music by Harry Dixon Loes.
19. Breneman, J. C., *Basics of Food Allergy* (Springfield, IL: Charles C. Thomas, 1978).
20. Crayhon, Robert, "The Paleolithic Diet and Its Modern Implications: An Interview with Loren Cordain, Ph.D.," www.chetday.com/cordaininterview.htm.
21. Budd, Martin, M.D., *Low Blood Sugar* (New York, NY: Sterling Publishing, 1981).
22. Kolata, Gina, "Questions Grow Over Usefulness of Some Routine Cancer Tests," *New York Times* 2001: Dec 30: A1–18. www.nytimes.com.
23. Kolata, A1–18.
24. *Citizens for Health Report* 2(1) (1994), www.citizens.org.

25. Colt, H. G. and Shapiro, A. G. "Drug-Induced Illness as a Cause for Admission to a Community Hospital." *Journal of the American Geriatrics Society* Vol 37 (1989), 323–26.

26. National Library of Medicine, "Allergic Rhinitis," www.nlm.nih.gov/medlineplus/ency/article/000813.htm. Accessed October 1, 2004.

27. *APUA Newletter* 19(2) (2001),2.

28. National Institute of Mental Health, "Antidepressant Medications," www.mental-health-matters.com/articles/nimh001.php?artID=236#ptdep7. Accessed October 5, 2004.

29. U.S. Department of Health and Human Services, "Over-the-Counter Drugs Aren't Risk Free," www.healthfinder.gov. Accessed October 2, 2004.

30. www.arthritis.com/nsaids.asp. Accessed October 2, 2004.

31. Mayo Clinic Staff, "NSAIDs: How to Avoid Side Effects," www.mayoclinic.com/invoke.cfm?objectid=E08D9F67-76D9-4D8F-B953CCEF9693D005. Accessed October 2, 2004.

Chapter Two

1. Murray, Michael T. *The Healing Power of Herbs: The Enlightened Person's Guide to the Wonders of Medicinal Plants, Second Edition* (Prima Publishing, 1992, 1995), 35.

2. Holt, Stephen, M.D., and Comac, Linda. *Miracle Herbs: How Herbs Combine with Modern Medicine to Treat Cancer, Heart Disease, AIDS, and More* (Carol Publishing Group, 1998), 94.

3. Holt and Comac, 94.

4. www.herbalgram.org, "Immunomodulating Compounds from Traditional Chinese Herbs."

5. Chang, Hson-Mou, Ph.D., and But, Paul Pui-Hay, Ph.D., eds., *Pharmacology and Applications of Chinese Materia Medica*

(World Scientific Publishing Co. Pte. Ltd., 1986, 1987), 1041.

6. Morazzoni, P., and Bombardelli, F., "Astragalus Root," *American Herbal Pharmacopoeia and Therapeutic Compendium* (Aug. 1999), 15.

7. Chu, D. T., et al., "Astragalus Root," *American Herbal Pharmacopoeia and Therapeutic Compendium* (Aug. 1999).

8. Zhang, Y. D., Shen, J. P. , Zhu, S. H., Huang, D. K., Ding, Y., Zhang, X. L. "Effects of astragalus (ASI, SK) on experimental liver injury." *Yaoxue Yuebao,* 1992 27(6): 401–6.

9. Mills, Simon, and Boone, Kerry, *Principles and Practice of Phytotherapy: Modern Herbal Medicine* (Harcourt Publishers Ltd., 2000), 315.

10. Fuchs, Nan Kathryn, *Modified Citrus Pectin (MCP): A Super Nutraceutica* (North Bergen, NJ: Basic Health Publications, 2003), 23.

11. Fuchs, 2.

12. Fuchs.

13. U.C. Davis Health System, "Breast Cancer,." http://www.ucdmc.ucdavis.edu/healthconsumers/health/000006.shtml.

14. Foster, Steven, and Chongxi, Yue, *Herbal Emissaries: Bringing Chinese Herbs to the West: A Guide to Gardening, Herbal Wisdom, and Well-Being* (Rochester, VT: Healing Arts Press, 1992), 61.

15. Lancet.1994 May7;343(8906):1122–6 http://www.ncbi.nlm.nih.gov/entrez/query.fcgi?cmd=Retrieve&db=PubMed&list_uids=7910230&dopt=Abstract

16. Hayakawa K., et al. Effect of Krestin (PSK) as adjuvant treatment on the prognosis after radical radiotherapy in patients with non-small cell lung cancer. Anticancer Research, 13:1815–1820(1993).

17. Holt and Comac, 91.
18. Carter, Joseph J., "Liver Protection and Repair: Synthesizing Herbal Science and Chinese Energetics," *Health Concerns Professional Newsletter* 3(1)4.
19. Foster and Chongxi, 76.
20. Foster and Chongxi ,213.
21. Subhuti Dharmandada, *Chinese Herbal Therapies for Immune Disorders* (Institute for Traditional Medicine and Preventative Health Care, 1988), 16.
22. Goldberg, Alice, and Brinckmann, Josef, eds., *Herbal Medicine* (Integrative Medicine Communications, 2000), 172.
23. McCaleb, Robert, et al., *The Encyclopedia of Popular Herbs: From the Herb Research Foundation, Your Complete Guide to the Leading Medicinal Plant* (Prima Lifestyles, 2000), 241.
24. McCaleb, et al., 243.
25. McCaleb, et al., 244.
26. Carper, Jean, "Eat Smart," *USA Weekend* (Nov. 16–18, 2001), 6.
27. www.nutritionaloutlook.com.
28. Murray, 194.
29. Murray, 194.
30. Chang and But, 712–16.
31. Chang and But, 712–16.
32. Chang and But, 712–16.
33. Chang and But, 712–16.
34. Jinhuang, Zhou, et al., eds., "Recent Advances in Chinese Herbal Drugs," *Science Press* 14 and *S.A.T.A.S.* (1991), 141–47.
35. Chang and But, 146.
36. *Journal of General Internal Medicine* (Jan. 2005 issue).
37. Scannell, Kate, M.D., "Medical Marijuana," *San Francisco Chronicle* (Feb. 16, 2003), D3.
38. Murray, 247.

39. Kupin, V., "Reishi Mushroom: Ganoderma Lucidum," *American Herbal Pharmacopoeia and Therapeutic Compendium* (Sept. 2000), 14.

40. Zhu-Fan, Xie, *Best of Traditional Chinese Medicine* (New World Press, 1995), 52.

41. Chang and But, 205.

42. Liu, G. T., "Pharmacological Actions and Clinical Uses of Fructus Schizandrae." in Zhou J., Liu, G. T., Chen, J., editor(s), *Recent Advances in Chinese Herbal Drugs—Actions and Uses* (Beijing: Science Press), p. 100–11

43. Brekman II, Dardymov IV, "New substances of plant origin which increase nonspecific resistance" *Ann Rev Pharm* 9:419–30

44. Sheldon, Saul, et al., eds., *PDR for Nutritional Supplements* (Medical Economics Company, Inc., 2001), 339.

45. Murray, 304.

46. Kirchheimer, Sid, "Soy Improves Prostate Cancer Outlook," http://my.webmd.com/content/article/94/102884.htm?z=3734_00000_1000_ts_02.

47. Murray, 296.

48. Chang and But, 494.

49. National Cancer Institute, "Antioxidants and Cancer Prevention," www.cancer.gov/cancertopics/factsheet/antioxidantsprevention.

50. Harvard School of Public Health, "Risk of Lung Cancer May Be Reduced by Eating a Wide Variety of Fruits and Vegetables," http://www.hsph.harvard.edu/press/releases/press10122000b.html.

51. Toniolo, P., et al., "Serum Carotenoids and Breast Cancer," *Am J Epidemiol* 153(12) (June 15, 2001), 1142–7.

52. Slattery, M. L., et al., "Carotenoids and Colon Cancer," *American Journal of Clinical Nutrition* 71(2) (Feb. 2000), 575–82.

53. Terry, P., et al., "Dietary Intake of Folic Acid and Colorectal Cancer Risk in a Cohort of Women," *Int J Cancer* 97(6) (Feb. 20, 2002), 864–67.

54. Emerson Ecologics, "Preventing Childhood Leukemia with Folic Acid," www.emersonecologics.com.

55. McCaleb, et al., 156.

56. Mayne, S. T., et al. Nutrient intake and risk of subtypes of esophageal and gastric cancer . *Cancer Epidemiol Biomarkers Prev.* 10:1055–62,2001.

57. Challem, Jack, "How to Save Your Skin," *Let's Live* (April 1999), 43.

58. *Alternative Therapies in Health and Medicine* 10(5) (Sept./Oct. 2004), 35. Mahon, B. D., et al., "Cytikine Profile in Patients with Multiple Sclerosis Following Vitamin D Supplementation," *J Neuoimmunol* 134(1–2) (2003), 128–32.

59. *Alternative Therapies in Health and Medicine* 10(5) (Sept./Oct. 2004), 35. Huisman, A. M., et al., "Vitamin D Levels in Women with Systemic Lupus Erythematosis and Fibromyalgia," *J. Rheumatol* 28(11) (2001), 2535–39.

60. *Alternative Therapies in Health and Medicine* 10(5) (Sept./Oct. 2004), 35. "Vitamin D Deficiency in the Morbidly Obese," *Obes Surg* (1993), 3, 421–24.

61. Alternative Therapies in Health and Medicine, 10(5) (Sept./Oct. 2004), 35. Grant, W. B., "An Estimate of Premature Cancer Mortality in the U.S. Due to Inadequate Doses of Solar Ultraviolet-B Radiation," *Cancer* 94(6) (2002), 1867–75.

62. Vasquez, D.C., N.D., Alex, Manso, M.D., Gilbert, Cannall, M.D., John. "The Clinical Importance of Vitamin D (Cholecalerferol): A Paradigm Shift with Implications for All Healthcare Providers," *Alternative Therapies in Health and Medicine* 10(5) (Sept./Oct. 2004), 33.

63. Jedrychowski, W., et al., "Nutrient Intake Patterns in Gastric and Colorectal Cancers," *Int J Occup Med Environ Health* 14(4) (2001), 391–95.
64. McCaleb, et al., 156.
65. Yance, Donald, and Valentine, Arlene, *Herbal Medicine, Healing & Cancer, First Edition* (McGraw-Hill, 1999), 197.
66. Pizzorno, Joseph E., Jr., and Murray, Michael T., eds., *Textbook of Natural Medicine, Second Edition* (Churchill Livingstone, 1993, 1999), 598.
67. Pizzorno and Murray
68. Challem, Jack, *The Inflammation Syndrome* (Hoboken, NJ: John Wiley & Sons, Inc., 2003), 109.
69. Chellem, 109.
70. Chellem, 107.
71. Sheldon, 201.
72. WholeHealthMD.com, "NAC (N-acetylcysteine)," http://www.wholehealthmd.com/refshelf/substances_ view/1,1525,809,00.html.
73. www.nutritionaloutlook.com.
74. Clark, L. C., et al., "Effects of Selenium Supplementation for Cancer Prevention in Patients with Carcinoma of the Skin," *JAMA* 276 (1996), 1957–63.
75. Yance and Valentine, 194.
76. Hu, Y-J, et al., "The Protective Role of Selenium on the Toxicity of Cisplatin-Contained Chemotherapy Regimen in Cancer Patients," *Biol Trace Elem Res* 56 (1997), 331–41.
77. Fawzi, Wafaie W.; Hunter, David J.; Kupka, Roland; Morris, Steve; Mugusi, Ferdinand; Msamanga, Gernard I.; and Spiegelman, Donna, "Selenium Status Is Associated with Accelerated HIV Disease Progression among HIV-1-Infected Pregnant Women in Tanzania," *J. Nutr* 134 (2004), 2556–60.

Chapter Three

1. NIDDK Office of Health Research Reports, "Addison's Disease: Adrenal Insufficiency," NIH Publication No. 04–3054 (June 2004), www.niddk.nih.gov/health/endo/pubs/addison/addison.htm.
2. www.alsa.org/.
3. Berkow, Robert, M.D., ed., *Merck Manual of Medical Information, Home Edition* (Pocket Books, 1997), 943.
4. Berkow, 868.
5. Suzuki, F., Kobayashi, M., Komatsu, Y., Kato, A., and Pollard, R. B. "*Keishi-ka-kei-to,* A Traditional Chinese Herbal Medicine Inhibits Pulmonary Metastasis of B16, Melanoma," *Anticancer Res* 17 (1997), 873–78.
6. www.WebMD.com.
7. Mayo Clinic Staff, "Chickenpox' (September 23,2004),
8. www.WebMD.com.
9. Carper, Jean, *Food:Your Miracle Medicine* (New York: HarperCollins, 1993), 43.
10. National Institute of Neurological Disorders and Stroke, "NINDS Guillain-Barre Syndrome Information Page,"
11. Nordenberg, Tamar, "Tossing and Turning No More: How to Get a Good Night's Sleep," *FDA Consumer* (July–August 1998), *www.fda.gov/fdac/features/1998/498_sleep.html.*
12. Brechka, Nicole, "Living with Lupus," *Let's Live* (October 2001), 60.

Chapter Five

1. Cascinu, S., et al., "Neuroprotective Effect of Reduced Glutathione on Oxaliplatin-Based Chemotherapy in Advanced Colorectal Cancer: A Randomized, Double-Blind, Placebo-Controlled Trial," *Journal of Clinical Oncology* 20 (2002), 3478–83.

Index

B

Backbone, 320
Bacteria, 15, 171
Ban lan gen, 138–39
Barley, pearl, 91
Basophils, 17
Baths, 40–41, 120
B cells, 17–18
Beliefs
  definition of, 59, 65
  limiting, 59–62
Benson, Herbert, 38–39
Bifidobacterium bifidum, 171
Biocidin, 320–21
Black walnut hulls, 321
Body, communicating with,
  55–56
Bone marrow, 16
Breathing, 94
Bronchitis, 190–92
Bupleurum, 124
Bupleurum Entangled Qi,
  321–22

C

Caffeine, 83–84
Calm Spirit, 322
Cancer, 192–201. *See also*
  Leukemia; Lymphoma
  case studies of, 197–201
  causes of, 195
  detection of, 193
  early warning signs of,
    194–95
  immune system and, 193
  lowering risk of, 195–96
  treatment of, 107–9, 193–94,
    196–97, 308–9, 310–11
Candida esophagitis, 201
Candidiasis, 202–10
  case studies of, 205–10
  chronic fatigue syndrome
    and, 218, 220
  symptoms of, 202
  tests for, 202

  treatment of, 202–5
Carotenes, 163–64
Catechins, 136
Caterpillar fungus, 126–27
Cat scratch fever, 210–11
Celiac disease, 80, 310
CFS. *See* Chronic fatigue
  syndrome
Chai hu, 124
Channel Flow, 322–23
Chemotherapy, 10, 107–9,
  307–8
Chickenpox, 211–13
Children, 119
Chinese medicine. *See* TCM
Chiropractors, 97
Chronic fatigue syndrome
  (CFS), 213–20
  candida overtreatment and,
    218, 220
  case studies of, 217–18, 220
  history of, 213–14
  symptoms of, 214
  treatment of, 215–16
Chronic lymphocytic leukemia
  (CLL), 243
Chronic myelocytic leukemia
  (CML), 243–44
Chuan xin lian, 121–22
Chzyme, 323
Ci wu jia, 131
Cirrhosis, primary biliary, 12
Citrus, 125
Clear Air, 323–24
Clear Heat, 324
Clearing, 325
Clear Phlegm, 324
CLL (chronic lymphocytic
  leukemia), 243
Cluster headaches, 229–30
CML (chronic myelocytic
  leukemia), 243–44
Codonopsis, 125–26
Coffee, 83–84
Cogni-Spark, 325

Books available
from Get Well Foundation

Healing Immune Disorders

by Andrew Gaeddert   ISBN 1-55643-604-1 $18.95

Healing Immune Disorders contains the latest scientific research on herbs and supplements and protocols for all major immune and autoimmune conditions. Whether you are a patient or a professional, you will be able to benefit from the advice in this book.

Healing Skin Disorders

by Andrew Gaeddert   ISBN 1-55643-452-9 $15.95

Filled with self-help strategies, treatment protocols, and case studies for all major skin disorders, this book is designed for the professional as well as the layperson. Dietary advice, acupuncture points, herbs, and nutritional supplements make this the most complete book of its kind.

Digestive Health NOW

by Andrew Gaeddert   ISBN 1-55643-426-6 $12.95

Digestive Health NOW explains a four-week program that can be completed in your home using a meal plan, recipes, and stress relieving techniques. Included are real-life stories of people who have been able to reduce or eliminate medication, and achieve an understanding of what causes symptoms and how to prevent them.

Healing Digestive Disorders, 2nd edition

by Andrew Gaeddert   ISBN 1-55643-508-8 $16.95

This book by herbalist Andrew Gaeddert lists self-help strategies, treatment protocols, and case studies for all major digestive disorders. Designed for the professional as well as the layperson, *Healing Digestive Disorders* also contains the story of how the author conquered Crohn's disease, a recommended meal plan, workbook section, and acupuncture points.

Chinese Herbs in the Western Clinic

by Andrew Gaeddert   ISBN 0-96382-850-9 $15.95

Chinese Herbs in the Western Clinic recommends formulas by variety of manufactures that have been successfully used by thousands of American patients. Disorders are alphabetized by Western conditions and indexed by traditional Chinese medical terminology for quick and easy reference. This book is designed for practitioners.

Sixty Years in Search of Cures

By Dr. Fung Fung
 and John Fung   ISBN 0-96382-851-7 $15.95

Sixty Years in Search of Cures is the autobiography of one of the world's most experienced herbalists, Dr. Fung Fung, who routinely saw 100 to 150 patients per day working in a hospital clinic. This master practitioner with experience in Canton, Hong Kong, Vietnam, and San Francisco, reveals important dietary and lifestyle habits for the general public and herbal prescriptions for the professional herbalist.

Send a check or money order payable to Get Well. Include $2.00 per book shipping and handling. California residents add 8.75% sales tax. Please write your name and address clearly, and specify the titles and quantities of each book you want. Allow 4 weeks for delivery.

For trade, bookstore and wholesale inquires, contact North Atlantic Books, P.O. Box 12327, Berkeley, CA 94701.

 Get Well Foundation
8001 Capwell Drive, Suite A
Oakland, CA 94621
Phone: 510-635-9778
Email: info@GetWellFoundation.org

About the Author

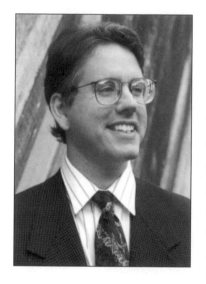

Andrew Gaeddert is one of the foremost herbalists and authorities on complementary treatments for immune disorders. Mr. Gaeddert has studied nutrition, herbology, and Chinese medicine with masters of herbal medicine in the United States and China. He has been on the protocol team of several scientific studies sponsored by the NIH Office of Alternative Medicine and the University of California of San Francisco, Canadian College of Oriental Medicine, and other colleges across the United States. His students have included medical doctors, acupuncturists, herbalists, and other professionals. Mr. Gaeddert is the author of *Healing Skin Disorders, Healing Digestive Disorders, 2nd edition, Digestive Health NOW,* and *Chinese Herbs in the Western Clinic,* and president of Health Concerns. He and his wife live in the San Francisco Bay area.